Prophylactic Mastectomy

Prophylactic Mastectomy

Insights from Women Who Chose to Reduce Their Risk

Andrea Farkas Patenaude, PhD

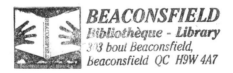

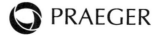 PRAEGER

AN IMPRINT OF ABC-CLIO, LLC
Santa Barbara, California • Denver, Colorado • Oxford, England

Library of Congress Cataloging-in-Publication Data

Patenaude, Andrea Farkas.
  Prophylactic mastectomy : insights from women who chose to reduce their risk / Andrea Farkas Patenaude.
    p. ; cm.
  Includes bibliographical references and index.
  ISBN 978–0–313–34516–6 (hardback : alk. paper) — ISBN 978–0–313–34517–3 (e–ISBN) I. Title.
  [DNLM: 1. Mastectomy—Autobiography. 2. Breast Neoplasms—prevention & control—Autobiography. 3. Decision Making—Autobiography. 4. Genetic Predisposition to Disease—psychology—Autobiography. 5. Genetic Testing—psychology—Autobiography. 6. Women—psychology—Autobiography. WP 910]
  616.99′44905900922—dc23   2011043403

ISBN: 978–0–313–34516–6
EISBN: 978–0–313–34517–3

16 15 14 13 12   1 2 3 4 5

This book is also available on the World Wide Web as an eBook.
Visit www.abc-clio.com for details.

Praeger
An Imprint of ABC-CLIO, LLC

ABC-CLIO, LLC
130 Cremona Drive, P.O. Box 1911
Santa Barbara, California 93116-1911

This book is printed on acid-free paper ∞

Manufactured in the United States of America

For Mason with love, pride, and hope
and
For all the women who generously shared their stories
and challenges with us

Contents

Preface

This book exists because I felt that what would be most helpful to women making decisions about prophylactic mastectomy (PM) was the voices of women who had already made the decision and had had surgery to remove their breasts in an effort to prevent cancer. This book contains narratives from interviews with 21 women who participated in a research study at the Dana-Farber Cancer Institute in Boston, Massachusetts. The research was supported by the U.S Army Research Materiel Command Breast Cancer Research Program under grant DAMD17-99-19162 and from grant 1 R03 HG003051 from the Ethical, Legal, and Social Implications Program of the National Human Genome Research Institute. The women were interviewed by either me or by Dr. Sara Orozco, another psychologist. The interviews took place by telephone after the woman read and signed a consent form about the nature of the research and the potential risks and benefits of being interviewed. The questions which were asked were based on clinical experience with women who had made or were considering this choice and from topics or dilemmas which had surfaced in the few articles in the literature. (See Appendix B for the list of interview questions we asked.) In Chapter 1, I describe the way we found the women we interviewed and elaborate on the interview process in greater detail

PM is not for everyone. Even if research were to show that PM could reduce to zero any risk of a woman's ever getting breast cancer (which it has not), it would not be acceptable to all women at high risk. Removing the breasts that might nurture one's children, excite one's partner, and add to one's sexual pleasure and feminine identification may just not be something many women are willing to do. However, the number of women undergoing PM is rising as the news of the success of this surgery for protecting high risk women becomes more solid and more widely disseminated. We will discuss in the chapters to come the factors influencing women's decisions, their experiences of surgery, and their assessments of the success of their choices on their quality of life.

This book can be used in a variety of ways. A woman in the process of deciding about whether or not she will have a PM may want to read the whole book, but not necessarily all at once. She may pick up and put down the book as her tolerance for hearing and thinking about PM waxes and wanes. She may want to give herself time to test out whether certain aspects of PM surgery are "for me." Others may want to read through the entire book to get an overview of the issues which women report about their experience or for hints about how to tackle making the decision. For some who know they want to have PM surgery, this book could even be seen as a reference guide to the points along the way and the issues which come up as PM surgery is accomplished and the period of adjustment begins.

Still, others who may not themselves be considering PM may see the chapters as stories of how women cope with a fascinating dilemma, choosing between living with significant cancer risk and living with a forever-changed body. The narratives may lead readers to challenge themselves by asking, "What would I be willing to give up to lower my risks of serious illness?" This question is one which many more people will be asking over the coming decades as more and more genes which predispose to other cancers and other serious illnesses are discovered.

Acknowledgments

This work would not have been possible without support from the Department of Defense Breast Cancer Program (Grant DAMD17-99-19162) and from the Ethical, Legal and Social Implications of the National Human Genome Research Institute (Grant 1 R03 HG003051). Special thanks are due to Dr. Elizabeth Thomson who saw the importance of this work and supported its completion.

I am deeply indebted to Dr. Sara Orozco who managed this research project, conducted the majority of the telephone interviews, interacted well with the physicians and with the women who were study subjects and, in general, kept this project running through difficult times.

I am grateful to Kelly Barrington, Sangetta Dey, Elizabeth Gagliardi, and Catherine Hoefliger for their thorough and sensitive coding of the interviews.

Surgeons at the Brigham and Women's, Massachusetts General, and Faulkner Hospitals in Boston were generous in encouraging this work and in allowing us to contact their patients to invite their participation, especially Drs. Michelle Gadd, Caroline Kaelin, Patricia Rae Kennedy, the late Yvette Matory, and Barbara Smith.

Dr. Judy Garber and Katherine Schneider M.P.H. helped to formulate issues to be addressed in this research.

Drs. Bob Weiss and Mary-Jo Good served as models of the value of qualitative research and the fact that books do get finished.

Drs. Michel Dorval, Martha Grootenhuis, Mary Jo Kupst, Susan Linn, Robert Noll, Susan Waisbren, and Lori Wiener have been supportive colleagues.

Drs. Ursula Matulonis, Michael Muto, Robert Ozols, Al Rabson, and Eric Winer contributed essentially to my ability to complete this book.

Larissa Hewitt, Michelle Cox, Barbara Keane, Martha Mahoney, and Peter Smith all contributed to the smooth running of this project and/or the preparation of the final manuscript, for which I am most grateful.

Debbie Carvalko and Praeger Publishers have been very patient and positive as they served as midwives to this project.

And, last, but most centrally, my love and thanks to Leonard whose belief in the importance of my work, support both practical and emotional, and loving kindness over many years has enabled me to tell this story.

Abbreviations

BRCA1/2 The breast cancer genes, BRCA1 and BRCA2, discovered in 1994 and 1995 which predispose female mutation carriers to high rates of breast and ovarian cancer, with the breast cancer often occurring at young ages.

DCIS Ductal carcinoma in situ. The most common form of non-invasive breast cancer. Has a high cure rate.

DIEP Deep Inferior Epigastric Perforator flap. A relatively new form of breast reconstruction in which only skin, fat, and blood vessels (but no muscles) are removed from other parts of the woman's body to be used in the construction of new breasts.

LCIS Lobular carcinoma in situ. A non-invasive accumulation of abnormal cells in the milk-producing (lobules) part of the breast. Not a true cancer, but should be watched as it is associated with increased risks for certain types of breast cancer.

PM Prophylactic mastectomy, surgical removal of the breasts of a woman in an effort to prevent breast cancer. Usually, PM is undertaken either by women known or suspected of having high hereditary risk for breast cancer who have not had breast cancer, or by women at high risk who have had cancer in one breast who have prophylactic removal of their other or contralateral breast to try to reduce their risk for a second breast cancer.

PO Prophylactic oophorectomy, surgical removal of the ovaries (and often also the Fallopian tubes and uterus) of a woman who has not had ovarian cancer but is at high hereditary risk to develop it, usually because she is a carrier of a *BRCA1/2* mutation or has a strong family history of ovarian cancer.

TRAM   Transverse Rectus Abdominis Muscle flap. A popular form of breast reconstruction involving surgical transposition of abdominal muscle as well as skin and fat to form the new breasts.

CHAPTER 1

Prophylactic Mastectomy: Is This for Me?

You really don't know. I wasn't prepared for physical feelings or emotional feelings, so you have to really explore and think about what you've heard other women experience and think, "Is that an issue for me? How would I react?" [Valerie]

For many centuries, cancer has been observed to occur more frequently than usual in certain families.[1] Within these families, members often lived with an expectation that the cancer which was so frequent among their family members would definitely occur sometime in their lives, generating considerable fear. Sometimes, it was not just one type of cancer, but several types, which ravaged family members. Until recently, there was little that could be done to manage that fear other than seeing a doctor regularly in hopes of finding the cancer early and having it removed before it had spread.

Many organs in the body are essential for life and hence, cannot be removed to prevent a cancer from occurring there and cannot be fully removed even if cancer occurs in that organ. Other body parts are routinely removed, either in part or in whole, when cancer is found. Surgery to remove breasts, ovaries, the colon, bones, kidneys, and other organs is common following a diagnosis of cancer. Mastectomies for breast cancer were the standard treatment until research published in the 1980s and 1990s showed that lumpectomies, removal only of the area containing and around the cancer, especially when paired with radiation therapy, might be equally effective in many cases.[2] Early mastectomies were termed "radical" and, indeed, that was what they seemed to be, often leaving the woman feeling quite disfigured and unable to resume full use of her arm on the side of the mastectomy.

It is not known who performed the first prophylactic mastectomy (PM), the surgical removal of healthy breasts from a woman at high risk of breast cancer, but they have been performed now for decades. Although still relatively rare, prophylactic mastectomies increased substantially following the advent of genetic testing for the *BRCA1/2* genes which identify the genetic mutations which predispose women to very high rates of breast and ovarian cancer.[3]

The *BRCA1/2* genes were found by looking at the DNA of men and women from families where the frequency of breast cancer was unusually high and often occurred at very early ages in women in the family. Scientists suspected that a genetic change or mutation might be responsible for the high number of cases of breast cancer in these families. In 1994, *BRCA1* was found,[4] quickly followed by the discovery of *BRCA2* in 1995.[5] These are powerful genes. Inheriting a gene from one parent who carries the deleterious (or bad) mutation conveys to a woman a lifetime risk of breast cancer of 56–85 percent,[6, 7] with the cancers often occurring at unusually young ages.[8, 9] To compare, the usual risk of breast cancer in the U.S. general population is estimated to be around 12 percent.[10] The *BRCA1/2* mutations can be inherited by men as well as by women and the children of mutation carriers have a 50/50 chance of inheriting the "bad" mutation from their parent, father or mother. Men who have a *BRCA2* mutation have a somewhat increased risk of developing breast cancer, but the risk is much lower than for women and it does not tend to occur at the early ages which characterize *BRCA1/2* mutation breast cancers in women. Men also may have slightly increased risks for prostate cancer.[11, 12]

It became clear that *BRCA1/2* mutations were also responsible for increased rates of cancer other than breast cancer in mutation carriers. The most frequent other cancer is ovarian cancer. Being a *BRCA1/2* mutation carrier raises the risk of ovarian cancer to as much as 40 percent. In the general U.S. population the risk is a little more than 1 percent among women.[10] There are also increased associated risks for pancreatic cancer for men and women mutation carriers,[11, 12] although these risks are much smaller than those for breast or ovarian cancer. Understanding how these genetic mutations work has helped us to know why some families suffered unusual amounts of cancer and cancer deaths. Because these are cancers that occur in adulthood, many of the individuals carrying these mutations had passed them on to their children before they themselves got sick, thus continuing the pattern of frequent cancers. It was also found that certain ethnic groups had particularly common *BRCA1/2* mutations due to early inbreeding among them in past centuries. Ashkenazi Jews and French-Canadians are just two ethnic groups with high rates of *BRCA1/2* mutations.[13, 14]

Once there was some understanding of the power of these two genes, the question of what could be done to reduce the risk of cancer in families which pass on the *BRCA1/2* mutations arose. With the knowledge of which specific genes were affected and the new scientific ability to sequence and look at genes to see if they have mutations, it was possible through this genetic sequencing or testing to discover which family members carry the deleterious mutations. After all, if the chances were 50/50 of inheriting a *BRCA1/2* mutation, this meant that half of the individuals in these families who were growing up fearing cancer did not have the mutation and would not have the unusually high risk of developing breast or ovarian cancer. (Individuals who are negative for a dominantly-inherited mutation (like *BRCA1/2* mutations) in their bloodline do still carry normal population level risks for breast and ovarian cancer; being negative on a *BRCA1/2* test does not guarantee that one will never get these cancers.)

For the other 50 percent who did inherit the deleterious mutation, the question was what should these mutation carriers do to detect these cancers early or, even ideally, to prevent the cancers from developing? Unfortunately, we do not yet have a commercially available "magic bullet" to simply turn off the *BRCA1/2* genes. This is an important goal which many scientists are working on, but, at present, the options are more limited and more complicated, all at once.

Many individuals in families with high rates of breast and ovarian cancer have come forward for genetic testing after the *BRCA1/2* genes were discovered in the mid-1990s. This is different from what occurred when the gene causing Huntington disease was discovered and many people from families with Huntington disease who had thought they would want to know if they carried the gene decided they did not want to know after all. Now, *BRCA1/2* testing is offered not just to members of known high risk families, but also often to women who are newly diagnosed with breast cancer, especially young women. These women are often tested immediately to see if they carry *BRCA1/2*, as it may affect the treatment they are given. More than 600,000 individuals (Rebecca Chambers, Myriad Genetics, personal communication. April 18, 2011) have been tested for *BRCA1/2*.

Guidelines were then developed, initially based solely on the opinion of experts, about what actions a woman with a *BRCA1/2* mutation might take to prevent or detect cancer. Even before the *BRCA1/2* genes were discovered, some of these recommendations had been given previously to members of high-risk families concerned about avoiding or finding breast cancer early in order to reduce the likelihood of a devastating cancer being found at a late stage, when treatment would not be successful or as successful.

The current recommendations, which have been refined as more research has been done over the past nearly 20 years, give women essentially two different paths to follow (sometimes sequentially) regarding their breast cancer risk. One path is a recommendation for early, frequent, and more involved screening for breast cancer. It is recommended that women begin breast screening at ages 25 or even earlier if the breast cancer in the family has been exceptionally early. It is also recommended that women have not only an annual mammogram, but also an annual breast MRI, as the latter can better detect some cancers. (Breast MRIs, however, have a high false positive rate, meaning that the MRI results often indicate there may be a cancer, when, with further testing, one is not found.) In addition to monthly breast self-exams (which some cancer treatment centers say women should start at age 18), the guidelines recommend that starting at ages 25, women have breast exams performed by a doctor twice a year. These actions are aimed at finding any breast cancer that might begin at a very early stage, when treatment is likely to be easier and more successful. Any woman who is at higher than usual risk of breast cancer due to her family history should consult a doctor to see if she should adopt these recommendations, whether or not she has had genetic testing. For women known to be mutation carriers, these recommendations are strongly encouraged.

The other path is one in which women are asked to consider surgery which might be able to prevent or drastically reduce the risk of breast cancer. Women who are mutation carriers for *BRCA1/2* are asked to think about whether they would be willing to have their breasts (or their ovaries, which we will discuss below) removed. Removing the breasts surgically was thought to be likely to vastly lower risks of developing breast cancer even before there was scientific data about the amount of risk reduction since the amount of remaining breast tissue is considerably reduced. Some breast tissue remains even with excellent surgery as it is difficult or impossible to take out all vulnerable tissue in the chest. Because doctors know that this is a major step for women to take, this surgery is not a "hard and fast" recommendation, even for mutation carriers, but rather something these women are asked to consider. Because doctors know that removing a woman's breasts might have significant psychological and interpersonal affects, they make sure to advise women to carefully consider this option.

A problem with this recommendation by physicians and surgeons is that it has often been difficult for both women considering surgery and their doctors to obtain information about how women feel when they undergo breast removal as a method of breast cancer prevention. There were few articles in the scientific literature and they did not offer very rich or detailed information about what it is like to make the decision about having a prophylactic mastectomy or to adjust to one's new body afterwards. These articles were scholarly in nature and not generally accessible to women in the general population. So, while women were told to think about prophylactic mastectomy, there was little or no guidance for them or their doctors about how to go about making this momentous decision. Some women were lucky enough to be connected to a woman who had already undergone this surgery and thus, were able to get some advice, but this was not always easy to arrange.

"Prophylactic mastectomy" was the term first used to describe the voluntary removal of one's breasts to try to prevent cancer. In recent years, some people have felt that the term "prophylactic" was misleading, since it is still possible for breast cancer to occur in the underlying tissues even after the breasts are removed. We have learned from research that the risk is small that this will happen (see the section below, "Does Prophylactic Mastectomy Work?"), but the possibility that one could still develop breast cancer is a consideration women have to factor into their decisions. Thus, some people felt that the term "risk-reducing mastectomy" would be more informative. I agree with this rationale. However, given that in the popular culture the term most used is "prophylactic mastectomy," I have chosen to use that term and its acronym "PM" throughout this book. I do hope that this is not construed by readers to assume that if they undergo PM surgery, their risks are reduced to zero of ever developing breast cancer. We will next describe in detail the research findings which tell how successful PM is in reducing risks for breast cancer.

In U.S.-based studies, the rate of uptake of PM among high risk women who have never had cancer is about 20–25 percent.[15, 16] Most of the subjects in these studies have been women who had genetic testing and knew they were carriers of *BRCA1/2* mutations. But, the majority of *BRCA1/2* mutation carriers are still opting not to undergo PM. They feel PM is just not for them or that the time is not right for this decision. Women who undergo PM tend to be in the period between ages 30 and 45.[15, 17] As the second generation of women who have known about *BRCA1/2* mutations comes of age, there are more young women learning about the option of PM and there may well be an increasing number who come to accept this surgical procedure. However, prophylactic mastectomy remains, as the authors of a recent meta-analysis (or overview of many reports) stated "a highly personal decision. Some women considering PM choose to live instead with a known risk of developing breast cancer."[18] We will discuss in the chapters to come how different women have different types of investment in their breasts, different ways of handling their breast cancer fear, and different approaches to managing their health risks.

DOES PROPHYLACTIC MASTECTOMY WORK?

Prophylactic mastectomy was performed even before there was hard evidence about its effectiveness. In the last part of the twentieth century and the early years of this century, studies were published which showed the efficacy of PM in reducing the risk of developing and dying from breast cancer. These were large and complex studies but they were not randomized, controlled trials, considered the gold standard in research, where each of two or more groups are randomly assigned a particular treatment or approach and the outcome measures are designed to optimize the likelihood of proving whether one treatment is clearly more effective. This is not possible for PM because women would not allow themselves to be randomly assigned to undergo a prophylactic mastectomy (or not).

The first of these studies on the effectiveness of PM was conducted at the Mayo Clinic in Minnesota.Dr. Lynn Hartmann and her colleagues showed that for high risk women who had not previously had breast cancer, having a PM reduced the woman's risk of developing breast cancer by 90–94 percent.[19] Among 639 women who had undergone a PM, seven women developed breast cancer after the surgery (all had had subcutaneous, and not a total mastectomy). This was less than half a percent of all the women who had had a PM. The women had been followed for a median of 14 years after their surgery. There were 214 women at high risk for breast cancer and 425 women at moderate risk of breast cancer in this group. The designation of being at either high or moderate risk was based on the woman's family history of breast and ovarian cancer. The 214 women at high risk were compared to their sisters; they had 403 sisters who had not had a PM.

Over the same period, 156 (38.7%) of the sisters of high risk women developed breast cancer while only three high risk women (about 1%) developed breast cancer. This was a reduction of 90–94 percent.

The risk of dying from breast cancer was also very substantially reduced for women who had undergone PM. Among the three high risk women who developed breast cancer after a PM, two died. Among the 156 sisters of these women who developed breast cancer, 90 died. Depending on the way the calculations of expected versus actual deaths are done, the risk of dying from breast cancer for a high risk woman who had had a PM was reduced 81–94 percent. For women at moderate risk, the statistics were even brighter. The rates of breast cancer in moderate risk women were compared to expected rates of breast cancer and of dying from this disease based on the Gail model of breast cancer risk.[20] The reduction of risk of developing breast cancer among the moderate risk women who had undergone PM compared to the rate at which they were expected to develop breast cancer (if they had not had a PM) was 89.5 percent. Women at moderate risk who had undergone PM also had a striking 100 percent reduction in their risk of dying from breast cancer. While the predicted incidence was that 10.4 of the 425 women would die of breast cancer without a PM, after having this surgery, none of the women in the group had died. An editorial accompanying th report of this Mayo Clinic study noted in speaking about the success of PM in reducing death from breast cancer, "It is difficult to think of a more effective strategy of cancer prevention."[21]

The second study detailing the positive effects of a prophylactic mastectomy was conducted in the Netherlands. Hanne Meijers-Heijboer and her colleagues reported on a group of 76 female *BRCA1/2* mutation carriers who had undergone bilateral (removal of both breasts) PM and been followed for an average of three years postsurgery.[22] They were compared with 63 women who had been tested at approximately the same time and were found also to be *BRCA1/2* mutation carriers, but who had elected not to undergo this surgery. Among the women in the PM group, there was a significant (p<0.003) reduction in breast cancer occurrence. In the PM group, no women developed breast cancer, while in the group which was being screened regularly for breast cancer but had not undergone PM, eight women developed breast cancer. Using a mathematical model based on these numbers, it was estimated that 2.5 percent of the women in the screening group who had not had a PM would be diagnosed with breast cancer each year and that nearly 25 percent would have breast cancer within 10 years.

The researchers estimated further that 35–50 percent of these women would die within 10–15 years of their diagnosis. In the *New England Journal of Medicine* editorial accompanying this study, the same authors who wrote the editorial for the Hartmann study concluded that, "Together, the studies by Meijers-Heijboer et al. and Hartmann et al. suggest that of the strategies to reduce the risk of breast cancer in high-risk women, prophylactic mastectomy is the most effective."[23]

Several other studies have also supported the very high reduction in breast cancer risk among women undergoing PM. Rebbeck and his colleagues[24] found a reduction of over 90 percent in a sample of women who were *BRCA1/2* mutation carriers. In this study, 102 of the mutation carriers had undergone PM and were followed for five years. In this PM group, two women developed breast cancer versus 184 of the 378 (48.7%) mutation carriers who had not had a PM. Another study by Ann Geiger et al.[25] of 276 women who had had a bilateral PM versus 196 randomly chosen women who had not had PM, showed that bilateral PM reduced the risk of developing breast cancer by 95 percent. Clearly, the effectiveness of a prophylactic mastectomy had been proven without a doubt by the results of these studies.

These studies also reinforced the feelings of women who had chosen to undergo PM before data was available to prove that it would substantially reduce their risk. The studies also gave physicians and surgeons firm ground for recommending PM to women at high risk by virtue of the breast and ovarian cancer in their family history. There was clearly medical benefit to PM. Many physicians had hesitated previously to recommend the removal of both breasts for women without a breast cancer diagnosis when women with breast cancer were being treated, at least in some parts of the United States, with lumpectomy, the removal of only the cancerous part of the breast. With this new strong data supporting the efficacy of PM, many more doctors began to talk more seriously to women about the consideration of PM since, as indicated by Eisen and Weber,[23] PM was a better cancer risk reducer than any other known intervention. There is, however, the continued recognition within the medical community that PM is not acceptable to all women and it remains a controversial intervention.[23]

WHO GETS PROPHYLACTIC MASTECTOMIES?

Among the estimated 200,000 women diagnosed with breast cancer in the United States this year,[26] approximately 5–10 percent or up to 20,000 women will have cancers attributable to hereditary muta-tions.[27] While many of the women who have *BRCA1/2* genetic testing and are found to be mutation carriers, or have uninformative results, will be asked to consider PM as a risk-reduction option, only a minor-ity will accept the surgery. For some women, it is a matter of time, with studies showing that many women take two years or more after learning they are mutation carriers to consider PM, before arranging to have surgery.[28] In a recent Danish study, the median time a woman had considered PM before surgery was over seven years after mutation testing.[3] In this study, only 11 percent had their PM surgery within six months of receiving a genetic test result.

Uptake rates of PM in the United States have ranged widely. In both U.S. and Canadian studies, uptake of PM has typically ranged from about 20–36 percent.[15, 16] Rates vary with the enthusiasm for PM of oncologists and surgeons in any particular area, although there are women in areas without a high uptake rate who have campaigned to have a PM based on personal judgment and strong internal motiva-tion. Uptake of PM does also vary significantly by country[15] with Dutch, Danish, and Belgian studies reporting the highest level of uptake, up to 50 percent in a recent Danish study.[3] Comparisons are difficult as the groups being considered sometimes include both women have never had breast cancer and those who are undergoing prophylactic mastectomy of the opposite breast after being diagnosed with cancer in the other breast. Some studies are limited to *BRCA1/2* mutation carriers, while some are not. Our focus will be on women without cancer who undergo PM, some doing so before there was genetic evidence that they were mutation carriers.

Not every woman who opts for PM has undergone genetic testing or has been found to be a mutation carrier. Among those who are tested, the majority of women who are genetically tested for *BRCA1/2* are given uninformative results, meaning that their family history does not clearly appear to be linked to *BRCA1/2*, at least at the level of our current understanding of which mutations are deleterious. Women with uninformative results are advised to follow screening regimens for those at high risk and they may choose to utilize PM to increase risk reduction. Some women decide on PM out of a strong breast cancer fear or frustration with multiple breast biopsies following equivocal mammograms, even without significant family history and without genetic testing. In one reported U.S. cohort of women undergoing PM, 37 percent had not had genetic testing prior to surgery.[29] This is likely to decrease as genetic testing becomes more common.

Women who decide to have a prophylactic mastectomy are noted in the literature to be more likely to:

- Be *BRCA1/2* mutation carriers[17]
- Have a sister with breast cancer[15]
- Be in their 30s or early 40s[3, 28, 30]
- Be divorced, widowed, or married[30]
- Have young children[3, 16, 28]
- Have high breast cancer distress and high risk perception[31, 32]
- Have had multiple breast biopsies[33]
- Have indicated before genetic testing that they would undergo PM[29, 34]

OUTCOMES OF PROPHYLACTIC MASTECTOMY

Given the clear message from the medical literature about the significant value of PM in reducing breast cancer diagnoses and deaths among women at high and moderate risk, especially among *BRCA1/2* mutation carriers, there has been increasing interest in finding how women who accept PM feel about their decision and about life after surgery. Physicians need this information to help inform patients considering PM. A number of articles have been published which address parts of these questions. Patients want this information to make informed decisions about PM and, for those women who have undergone PM, to compare their own experience to that of others. We will briefly summarize what has been reported in the medical and psychological literature about outcomes of PM.

Satisfaction with Their Decision

Generally, women who have chosen to undergo PM have later reported being very satisfied with their decision. Few—0 percent to 19 percent—expressed regret or dissatisfaction with their decision.[35, 36, 37, 38, 39, 40, 41, 42] Critics have wondered if the lack of expressed regret among women who have undergone PM might be due to the fact that it would be very difficult emotionally to believe one had made a mistake in such a major decision. It would also be difficult to express this publicly, especially when there might have been, as was often the case, opposition in one's family or even among one's medical providers early on about PM. On the other hand, the consistency of this finding in widely separated samples over time suggests that, in fact, most women who have a PM are genuinely relieved about reducing what had felt like a potentially consuming breast cancer risk and they do not regret their decision.

For women without cancer, the choice of reconstructive surgery is not constrained by considerations of future treatment; the timing is elective and there is a longer period over which to gain information about prophylactic mastectomy and to consider the options. Hence, satisfaction rates tend to be somewhat higher among women with bilateral prophylactic mastectomy who did not have breast cancer. However, satisfaction with reconstruction is lower than with the decision to have a PM.[37] As we shall see in later chapters, being satisfied with the overall decision does not mean that women do not have complaints about the length or nature of the PM experience.

Complications of PM

Complication rates are high in prophylactic mastectomies, although rates are lower among unaffected women undergoing bilateral mastectomy than for women with cancer who are having prophylactic removal of the contralateral (other side) breast.[42]

Complication rates vary by procedure, by whether or not the woman has had cancer or has other medical conditions, and by location and surgeon. Thus, it may be difficult to interpret published rates, which can seem very high. Studies are also difficult to compare because of differences in the definition of "complication" and differences in the type of medical procedure being undertaken. There is some indication that more recent surgeries are actually more complicated surgically and, thus, may have higher complication rates.[43] A 2005 study of 269 women from six healthcare plans across the United States who had no personal history of breast cancer were followed for an average of seven years postsurgery.[44] Eighty percent had reconstruction, most of which were implants. One or more complications occurred in 64 percent of the female patients following surgery; the average woman who had reconstruction had 2–2.4 complications per patient. These complications included pain (35%), infection (17%), and seroma or drainage of lymphatic fluid in 17 percent of cases. Women without reconstruction had fewer complications. Those who had later reconstruction (not at the same time as the mastectomy surgery) had slightly higher rates of complications. Most of the complications occurred within a month of surgery; half of the incidents of pain noted occurred within 10 days of surgery, although in some cases, the pain persisted for years. About a quarter of the patients had an unanticipated surgery as part of the reconstruction effort.

A study which reported on 55 cases of Deep Inferior Epigastric Perforator (DIEP) flap reconstruction in a group of mixed cancer patients and unaffected women undergoing bilateral PM showed that, in about 13 percent of the cases, there was necrosis or death of the tissues in the flap.[45] A hematoma (or semisolid blood mass) formed under the flap in 7.2 percent of cases, necessitating surgical re-operation and in 7.2 percent of cases, transfusion was necessary because of excessive blood loss. The authors of this study feel this represented an acceptable level of complication; 96.2 percent of patients said they would recommend the procedure to their friends if they were in the same position.

These findings are presented only as an indication of what complications might occur and to highlight the fact that complications are not rare in PM. This can serve as a guide for women to initiate conversation with surgeons about the nature and frequency of the complications which they have seen with the type or types of reconstruction being considered. In future chapters, we will discuss women's experience of these complications to broaden our understanding of the impact of complications on a woman's quality of life.

Reduction in Cancer Worry

It has been found that having a prophylactic mastectomy greatly reduces worry about developing breast cancer.[41, 46, 47, 48] Many studies show significant declines in rates of anxiety and cancer-related worries following prophylactic mastectomy for most women.[38, 46] Perception of risk for breast cancer is also typically strongly decreased following PM.[49] Clearly, PM is successful in this regard; most women feel strongly that by undergoing surgery, they have significantly reduced their heightened breast cancer risk. While some women do continue to worry, studies suggest that this is related to high initial worry, which may reflect a personality variable.[31]

Body Image and Sexuality

Many women do report negative changes in their body image after prophylactic mastectomy. A recent Swedish study reported that the importance of the breasts was reduced in 69 percent of the 59 women with no history of breast cancer who had undergone PM and 75 percent felt their sexual enjoyment changed in a negative way after PM.[50] There was considerable individual variation in whether these women felt that sexual intercourse and their own sense of sexual attractiveness had changed after PM. An earlier study found 44 percent of women felt that PM had adversely affected their sexual relationship.[37] However, a U.S. study found the majority of women post–PM reported no change in their self-esteem, sexual relationships, or feelings of femininity.[38] In that study, 36 percent of the women reported diminished or greatly diminished satisfaction with their appearance after PM, 25 percent reported diminished feelings of femininity, and 23 percent said their sexual relationship had been adversely affected. Interestingly, there have been reports of improved sexual functioning as well after PM.[37] We will report in depth on the body image, sexual attractiveness, and sexual functioning of post-PM women in our study in Chapter 6.

Overall Quality of Life

Studies of quality of life after prophylactic mastectomy are difficult to evaluate and compare. Many studies mix subjects with and without a personal cancer history, making differentiation difficult of what is specifically the impact of the surgery. There is surgery-associated distress and, as we have just discussed, an impact on both body image and sense of sexual attractiveness for many women and an impaired quality of life, at least temporarily, in some studies.[51] Nonetheless, women often report little negative change in their overall quality of life[52] and reports of sexual functioning after surgery are mixed[38, 53] with some women reporting more enjoyment of sex as a result of feeling less worried about cancer and dying. Major disruption in quality of life does not seem to be typical after surgery, but it is clear that recovery is complex and takes months and, in some cases, even longer. As we shall discuss in more detail in other chapters of this book, women adjusting to life after PM can nearly simultaneously experience both positive and negative reactions.

RECONSTRUCTION OPTIONS

This is not a book about the currently available options for breast reconstruction; that book would be best written by surgeons and plastic surgeons. To summarize, there are two main types of reconstruction,

those that utilize fat and other tissue from other parts of the woman's
body (and are sometimes referred to as "autologous" procedures
involving "flaps") and those that create spaces into which implants can
be inserted. The options open to women for reconstruction change
with advancing surgical techniques, with social acceptance of implant
materials, and with preferences and trade-offs which women are willing
to accept at different points in time and in different geographic loca-
tions. For example, in the last decade or so, it was felt that total mastectomies which did not leave nipples intact were the most beneficial, as
they left the least amount of residual tissues in which breast cancer
could develop. More recently, partially because of women's unhappiness about losing their nipples for cosmetic (i.e., appearance) reasons
and for the sensation which an intact nipple can convey and partially
because of improved technique, some surgeons are now reconsidering
nipple-sparing mastectomies.[54] Another emerging technique is the
Deep Inferior Epigastric Perforator flap, often referred to as DIEP,
which is currently gaining favor compared to the TRAM (Transverse
Rectus Abdominis Myocutaneous) flap, the "current mainstay in choice
of autologous reconstruction."[55] There is, however, no completely
"free lunch" in breast reconstruction. The DIEP technique reduces
the risk of some complications, but has disadvantages in terms of certain other types of complications.[56]

There have also been changes in the types of implants used over
time. Saline has been used since silicone implants were banned in the
United States in 1996. However, in 2006, silicone implants, which
have undergone technological improvements, were again approved
and are now seen by some as offering advantages.[57] However, no form
of reconstruction is without potential complication and there are
often reasons why additional, unplanned surgeries are needed in the
process of completing the reconstruction.

What is clear is that women need to talk at length to surgeons and
plastic surgeons in their community to discover what options for
breast reconstruction are available locally. Not all techniques work
with all body types. Habits, like smoking, may make some procedures
less likely to succeed than others for a particular woman. Thus,
women who want breast reconstruction have to discover—perhaps
from talking to several surgeons—what their body type and history
can best support. In thinking about relatively new techniques, women
may want to inquire about how many such surgeries the surgeon or
plastic surgeon has performed and if there are other surgeons who
have more experience. (Breast surgeons typically remove the breasts

and plastic surgeons are present to initiate the reconstructive part of the surgery.) Whether or not surgery in a distant city is an option can vary. Some women will travel anywhere and others feel they would not have surgery anywhere but close to home. Many of the women in our study spoke to many surgeons and plastic surgeons and found these discussions to be useful. In this study and elsewhere,[58] women also found it helpful to view photographs of the surgeon's prior reconstructions or photos p comparing reconstruction outcomes using different techniques.

It is also true that surgeons may not be able to determine their ability to utilize a particular reconstructive technique until they begin the operation,[59] so it is important to discuss what the fallback position is if they are not able to do the intended surgery. PM surgeries tend to be long surgeries; two studies repeated mean times of 9.3 hours with a range of 3 to 16 hours[60] and a mean of 8 hours with a range from 6 hours and 38 minutes to 16 hours.[45] Knowing this in advance may allay fears for the waiting family and for the patient when she awakens from the procedure.

Readers are, therefore, referred to their own physicians, surgeons, and plastic surgeons who can provide current information about the types of reconstruction available in their area and elsewhere and about the particulars of the anticipated surgery. If you do not know how to find a breast surgeon or plastic surgeon, talk to your family doctor or internist or contact the local hospital's oncology or breast oncology department. Feel free to ask questions and to ask for printed materials about the type of surgery that is being recommended. You can also ask to speak to previous patients of the surgeon who have undergone the recommended procedure.

SUMMARY

Prophylactic mastectomy (PM) is an established technique for the reduction of breast cancer occurrence in women at high hereditary risk. With more than 600,000 women tested for *BRCA1/2* in the United States, there will be many women considering PM in the next decades. While we now have data suggesting who chooses PM and, in general,[61] what types of outcomes, positive and negative, these women experience, we hope that the narratives reported in the chapters to come will illustrate the dilemmas faced by women in this circumstance and what it has meant to them emotionally and interpersonally to choose PM as their way to reduce high risks for breast cancer. Our study, which we will describe in the next section, provides the opportunity to read—in the women's own words—about the issues which motivated this sample of 21 women to choose PM, their experience of surgery, and the adjustments, problems, satisfactions, and triumphs which they spoke of in our interviews.

THIS STUDY

The book offers a rich description of the process of making a decision about prophylactic mastectomy, having PM surgery, and adjusting to life after this surgery. The path is guided by narratives taken from interviews conducted with 21 women who have undergone PM. These women have never had breast cancer but their family history, sometimes coupled with other events, made them feel PM was the right answer for them to minimize their breast cancer risk and allay their fears. They came to PM in different ways; they had different life histories and experiences. Many of their worries and feelings about breast cancer, however, were the same: that it was a "tiger on their trail" that had previously laid prey to some of their family members. The women were searching for a way to change the course of their family history and, in so doing, relieve themselves of the worry about breast cancer and the sense of its imminence, which they often felt.

These interviews were undertaken as part of a larger study about psychological issues related to prophylactic mastectomy which was funded by the U.S. Department of Defense Breast Cancer Program and the Ethical, Legal, and Social Implications Program of the U.S. National Human Genome Research Institute. The interviews were conducted by a psychologist via telephone and were recorded, transcribed, and coded. These women had had bilateral prophylactic mastectomies at one of several Boston hospitals in the Harvard system (Brigham and Women's Hospital, Massachusetts General Hospital, or Faulkner Hospital). The women had to be at least one year beyond their surgery to be eligible for the study. In addition, they had to speak English sufficiently well enough to participate in a telephone interview.

Actual study participation required (1) completion of a mailed questionnaire about the woman's demographic characteristics (age, education, marital and childbearing status, income, and occupation), surgical information, and family history and (2) participation in one telephone interview. Informed consent was evidenced by the signing of a consent form approved by the Dana-Farber Cancer Institute Institutional Review Board and the Human Subjects Research Review Board of the U.S. Army Medical Research and Materiel Command. Subjects received $25 for their participation in this study.

Women who had undergone a PM since 1990 who had never developed breast cancer or ductal carcinoma in situ (DCIS) were identified from medical records at the participating hospitals. Surgeons whose patients were identified were contacted to verify that the mastectomy they had preformed was a prophylactic mastectomy and to request permission to send the woman a letter inviting her to participate in this study. Permission to contact their patients was granted by 97 percent of the 33 surgeons we contacted. Surgeons also agreed to sign a letter about study participation which was sent to the eligible women, as it was felt that it would be more comfortable for women to learn of their study through their own doctor. Three surgeons preferred that we contact patients directly and, in those cases, the letter came from the project principal investigator. With the original letter, we sent an opt-out card which women not wishing to participate in the study could return and not be contacted further. If that card was not returned within two weeks, the study coordinator contacted the eligible woman, described the study further and, if the woman was willing, asked her to sign and return the consent form and the questionnaire. The interview was scheduled at the convenience of the subject. Eighty percent of the women we invited agreed to participate in the study.

The interview was semi-structured and the interviewers encouraged subjects to answer questions as fully as they wished. If short or incomplete answers were given, interviewers were trained to ask probing questions to encourage detailed responses. The interview focused on the woman's motivation for having a PM and the process by which she came to her decision including her communication with medical providers and relatives about PM. It also focused on her surgical and reconstructive experiences, the physical aftereffects the woman experienced, and on her emotional adaptation to her changed body. We asked about the impact on her body image and sense of physical attractiveness and on whether there had been significant changes in her sexual functioning and the interpersonal relationship with her significant other, if she had one. We asked about satisfactions and regrets and her communication about PM with family members, co-workers, and friends. We also inquired about whether she had had psychological consultation and/or consultation with other women who had had PM. If so, we asked if these consultations had been useful or could be useful to others who were considering PM. The interview questions are available in Appendix B of this book.

The women who were interviewed seemed in general to talk readily and conversationally about their experiences. It seemed that many were glad to have a reason to tell someone else in detail about their experiences. Many expressed a wish to help others and offered to be peer counselors for women considering PM if the need arose. The average length of the interviews was 53 minutes.

Characteristics of the Participants

The mean age of the women we interviewed who had not had breast cancer and had undergone bilateral prophylactic mastectomy was 45.4 years old, with a range from 32 to 62 years (see Appendix A for demographics of participants). All but one (95%) were married and 86 percent had children at the time we interviewed them. Ninety percent of the women identified as Caucasian; one said she was Native American and another listed her race as "Other." This was a well-educated group of women, with 72 percent having a college degree or further graduate study. Over half said their family income was more than $100,000. Forty-eight percent were employed full time and about a quarter of the total sample was employed in the health professions.

The average age of the women at the time of their surgery was 40.1 years with a range from 29 to 52 years. The women were an average of 5.2 years beyond their surgery at the time of their interviews. None of the women had ever developed breast or ovarian cancer. One woman developed lobular carcinoma in situ (LCIS) after her PM. Fifteen out of the 21 women (71%) rated their current health as excellent or very good.

Among the 21 women in our study, 19 had mothers who had developed breast cancer. In 11 cases, the mother had developed breast cancer before she was 50 years old. Sixteen of the women had mothers who had died of breast cancer; the average age of the mother at her death was 54.4 years. Five of the women (24%) had been under age 18 when their mother died. Nine women (43%) had at least one sister who had had breast cancer, with two women having three affected (i.e., having had cancer) sisters and one woman having two affected sisters. Seven women (33%) had a grandmother who had developed breast cancer; all were maternal grandmothers except one. Four women (19%) had a first or second degree relative who had had ovarian cancer. Five women had a father, grandfather, or uncle with prostate cancer (24%). Three knew they carried a hereditary breast cancer mutation in their families, one knew she did not have a familial mutation, one preferred not to say, and most did not know if there was a hereditary breast cancer disposing mutation in their family.

What Did We Want to Know?

We were guided in what we wanted to know by both interviews which we conducted in another part of the project with 37 women who were currently considering prophylactic mastectomy and from our assessment of the gaps in the existing literature about PM. While many questions women have are about the technical aspects of the surgical and reconstruction options that exist, many of those questions can be answered by their surgeons and plastic surgeons. Our focus was on the emotional aspects of what women wanted to know about the PM experience. What could we tell them about other women's experiences that would make the decision about PM and, if they chose surgery, the preparation for and adjustment to surgery, better for them?

The women considering PM told us they were eager to know how others had made their decision about PM. How had they had contacted the doctors they needed to contact and how had they decided on one technique versus another? They were also eager to know whether women had talked to their husbands or partners about the surgery and what was discussed. Did sexual partners find it more difficult after surgery than they thought they would to deal with the woman's changed body? Were these partners rejecting or sexually less interested? How did the women themselves feel about their changed bodies? Did the women find it harder than they had anticipated? Did they feel that they were "less of a woman"? How long did it take for the woman to feel better after surgery? Did she ever feel "normal" again?

These women also wanted to know how had other family members reacted. How had the women talked to their children about PM and when? How did the children react, especially the adolescent girls? Did the children find it traumatic for their mother to have this surgery? To what degree did it bring up issues about breast cancer and prior losses in families which were difficult to deal with?

How did PM interfere with a woman's ability to play sports as she had before? How long did it take to be able to get back to playing the sport? Will one feel comfortable in a locker room changing clothes?

How does one contact a woman who has undergone a PM? Who does one tell and how much does one say about this surgery? Do people stare? How did the woman handle it at work? Does one tell people what kind of surgery and why or why not? Are people helpful or insensitive? How to handle the insensitive questions about why one is having such a "barbaric thing" done to her body?

How much detail did the woman have before surgery about what it would really be like? How different is the surgical experience for different women? What if complications occur? Are complications common?

Do women regret their decision? How do the breasts look and feel? Do the women find the peace of mind they were seeking and feel better afterwards and not worry so much about breast cancer? How do women feel about their new breasts if they have reconstruction? Do the new breasts come to feel like part of the woman's body or not?

We shall explore answers to these questions from the narratives of the women we interviewed. Their words detail the experiences they had and their satisfactions and dissatisfactions with aspects of their experiences. These women are pioneers in undergoing prophylactic mastectomy and they were eager to share what they knew with other women, to try to make things easier for those who came after them.

CHAPTER 2

Motivation for Prophylactic Mastectomy

It is fear of getting breast cancer that motivates most women to consider surgical removal of healthy breasts. However, within that motive, there are many more specific feelings which underlie the equation that leads a particular woman to this conclusion. "I felt that I was in a room and there was only one door," was one woman's description of the feeling which dominated her decision making. Many professionals and lay people alike have considered prophylactic masectomy (PM) to be overkill, to be unacceptable, as reflected in the 2005 article title about women's attitudes towards PM.,[1] "That's like chopping off a finger because you're afraid it might get broken: Disease and illness in women's views of prophylactic mastectomy." However, an increasing number of women are making a decision for PM when faced with the knowledge that they have a greatly increased risk for breast cancer on the basis of their family history and/or because they are found, through genetic testing, to be carriers of mutations in a high-risk cancer gene. This chapter describes the motivations of 21 women who underwent PM without having had breast cancer out of a fear that they were very likely to get breast cancer.

NOT YOUR MOTHER'S BREAST CANCER: THE MOTIVATING INFLUENCE OF FAMILY EXPERIENCE

Perhaps the strongest motivation for undergoing a prophylactic mastectomy among women we interviewed was having experienced the illness, treatment, and death of a mother from breast cancer. Seventy-six percent of the women in our study who had undergone bilateral PM had mothers who died of breast cancer, 29 percent of them before she, the daughter, was 21 years old. While it is true that not everyone whose mother has been diagnosed with breast cancer chooses PM, having had an ill mother is clearly an early and powerful lesson that cancer is a devastating disease. Many of the women in our study talked about this powerful influence. They talked about deciding at the time of their mother's illness that they would do everything they could to avoid finding themselves ill with cancer at an early age.

Beth's (all names are fictional) experience certainly exemplified this thinking. She came from four generations of Ashkenazi Jewish women who had died of breast cancer. Beth was one of four sisters. Her mother was diagnosed with breast cancer when Beth was 18 years old. By the time Beth was 20 years old, her mother had "made" her get a baseline mammogram. Beth's mother told her four daughters, "If there's the chance and you guys can do it surgically, just cut them off." Beth describes herself and her sisters as having been "preconditioned to not having our breasts for a long time." Her parents took very active steps to try to get their daughters the best possible medical information. In her late twenties, Beth and her family participated in a research project to discover the first breast cancer gene. She was told that she and one of her sisters had genetic markers which were the same as her mother's, with the implication that she likely carried the family's predisposition to breast cancer. At age 33, after having her second child, Beth followed her mother's advice and underwent a bilateral prophylactic mastectomy.

Another woman, Meredith, stated, "I've known since I was twenty that I was going to do it . . . I'd much rather do that than watch what my mother went through." Meredith begins her story:

> Well, I had just buried my mother and about two months later, I read about it [prophylactic mastectomy] . . . When I was 21, even then, it seemed like not something I wanted to do right then and there, but something that I wanted to do after I'd had my kids and was closer to the age of forty. But I never thought I was going to be able to because at that time it wasn't something that insurance would cover. Then later on, I came into an inheritance and I actually wanted to pay for it myself, but my doctor said, "I think actually insurance is paying for it now if you qualify."

Some of Meredith's desire to undergo PM may have been the result of an interaction with a physician who was taking care of her mother. Around the age of 18, Meredith had accompanied her mother to an office visit in Boston for treatment. The doctor, who had a daughter about the same age, reportedly asked to see her.

He told me that my mother had, I forget what he called it, but it was an extremely aggressive form [of cancer]. Like they had found hers when it was only a pinpoint, not even a lump. Her nipple had inverted, and all they could find was like a tiny pencil point when they were doing frozen sections. Even at that point, it had spread to her lungs and throughout her body. Although she survived, maybe like from the age of five until I was 21, she was constantly in and out of hospitals. He told me hers was extremely aggressive and hormone driven and even then he said it appears to run in families, although they didn't know much about it then. He told me, he came right out and told me to enjoy my life because in all likelihood it might not be a very long one!

After her mother's death, Meredith was careful to take good physical care of herself and to be screened regularly for cancer. At 25, she "went to the doctor hysterical about a lump" she had felt in her breast. It did not turn out to be breast cancer, but after that she had regular clinical breast exams. She later felt another "obvious hard lump in my breast. So I went to the doctor and the doctor, of course, with my family history, freaked out and thought I had a tumor. No one thought to give me a pregnancy test." Instead, Meredith underwent tests involving radiation. "It turned out I was pregnant and the radiation did affect the fetus, so I lost the baby. It was a blocked milk duct."

When Meredith was pregnant with her second child, she discovered another hard lump in her breast and had a biopsy done with only local anesthesia. Iit turned out to be another blocked milk duct. These cumulative experiences nonetheless convinced Meredith that when she was finished having her children, she would undergo a prophylactic mastectomy. After her second child was born, Meredith said she "started having trouble sleeping at night because I was thinking, 'God, I'm the same age. She [her mother] was thirty-five when she had me and I'm thirty-six. I've got this little baby, and you know, the next thing you know, I'm forty.' I kept thinking forty-one is coming and I've got to do something before that." She carefully planned to have the surgery when her second child reached the age of 3 when it would not, she thought, be so difficult for him to be sent away to relatives for a few weeks as she recovered. At 39, she finally had the surgery she had been thinking of since she was 21.

The surgery has not taken away all of Meredith's cancer fears, but it allows her to "have a better shot at seeing my grandchildren." She knows there is some residual risk.

> Yes, I just didn't want my kids going through it. Like I know what it's like, and I just wanted my kids to—even if I do, because I still have—there's still a chance. There's breast tissue in your ribs that they can't get rid of, and there's still a chance that you can get it. But, I mean, even if I get it when they're in their twenties, they're grown up then and they didn't grow up with it. They're on their own.

Sometimes the decision for PM follows the diagnosis of breast cancer in a sister or other relative. The effects are clearly cumulative, so that when one or more family members develops cancer, even if they are not all breast cancers, the fear of cancer becomes more prominent and the push towards surgery intensifies. Janice dates her decision to a period when she was:

> starting approaching thirty-five, because my mother had had it, and her mother had had it, both at thirty-five and died at thirty-seven of breast cancer. Then my son got diagnosed at the age of three with a brain tumor, but it was a benign brain tumor. It's [PM] just something that's been there through the years. Then my younger sister got diagnosed with breast cancer, and then, bingo, everything just started to fall into place. Then with the cyst we were following, I said, "With everything happening this's just something I just had to try to think about" and I knew that that [PM] was the decision I had to make.

CANCER IS COMING

A residual effect of watching a mother, sister, grandmother, or multiple family members sicken and often die of a cancer is that it begins to feel inevitable that the younger generation will also fall victim to cancer. Many of the women who opted for bilateral prophylactic mastectomy spoke with passion about the feeling that breast cancer was "coming." This was not about the hypothetical concept of risk, of chances that one might or might not develop cancer. This was the certainty that it was coming and it was only a matter of time. Some women literally talked of trying to outrun the disease without getting caught; not "if" but "when" was the only question. This presumed "ribbon of fate" connected those not yet affected by disease with their affected and often deceased ancestors; what had happened would happen again. Such vulnerability was a function of membership in their family. These women considered prophylactic mastectomy in light of their perception of the inevitability of getting sick.

> It was just something I kind of took for granted. It was like, "I know it's going to happen" sort of thing. [Alice]
>
> My husband and I sort of felt like it's the best thing to do because I'm pretty much predestined for a disease and this way we can control it. I think ___ (my husband) said to me, "Better to be proactive than reactive." [Beth]

Phrases like "ticking time bomb" or "Russian Roulette" signified an approaching encounter with the fate which had previously engulfed the lives of other relatives. Kate said that:

> I was under the care of a breast specialist out of the Brigham and Women's Hospital. I felt like I was in such good hands because they had seen all of this, and just felt that I was a ticking time bomb and I needed to do something. . . . Given my strong family history and just watching what my sister had gone through, I just knew it was only a matter of time. That's kind of how I lived my whole life at that point, of just waiting to find it.

Joyce told us, "I guess my feeling was that I was playing Russian Roulette and that I needed to go see somebody." She went on, "I remember reading an article about this in *Newsweek* magazine and somebody in a similar position said she felt like she had 'two loaded revolvers pointed at her chest.' I remember reading that and thinking, 'That's exactly like how I feel.'"

For some women, genetics was clearly the "ribbon of fate" connecting bad past experience to the inevitability of their own illness. Janice described thinking, "If I didn't have it [PM], I'd probably end up with breast cancer. I definitely would, because I do have the genes." The sporadic but unrelenting cancer diagnoses of other relatives felt like a harbinger of things to come. Laura told us, "It's not something

I think about every day or I would even say every week, but there were times when I would hear about other family members or just have a sense of foreboding, how long do I have?" Another unaffected woman, however, described feeling as if she already did have cancer based on her worry. Kate said, "I felt like I had it already somehow, crazy as that sounds. That was a horrible way to live your life."

While the inevitable diagnosis of cancer seemed to be a given, some women believed that the knowledge they had gained about how to care for themselves might alter the outcome, and thus might give them more hope of surviving the cancer than had been the case for their mother, aunt, sister, etc. Julia said, "I always felt if I got it, I'd get it [i.e. catch it] early, and it wasn't going to be a problem. It was kind of like I felt like I'd always get breast cancer, but I took care of myself, so I'd always get it early. I'd get the monthly checks and so I never really thought it would kill me."

In other families where mastectomies had been the way other women had dealt with their disease, prophylactic mastectomy also sometimes seemed inevitable. In Beth's family, "It was pretty obvious that we weren't going to—either we weren't going to be around for a long time or we weren't going to have them [breasts] for a long time. Everyone in my family had bilateral full mastectomies."

IMPACT OF REPEATED BIOPSIES OR OTHER MEDICAL SCARES ON THE DECISION FOR PM

Many women trace at least the final step in their decision to undergo PM to fear and frustration associated with repeated medical near-misses. These too-close-for-comfort events were, for some women, the need to undergo mammograms with many extra films, and, for other women, the discovery and investigation of cysts and/or the experience of undergoing multiple biopsies. The cumulative worry, the repeated experience of having doctors or technicians suggest that something might not be right within their breasts, led these women to take the step of scheduling their PM surgery. This felt like a way out of what the women experienced as a lack of control, a hell of sorts where they could be held hostage by their cancer fear, sometimes for extended periods, as efforts were made to work up a suspicious lump or shadow. The decision for PM is therefore described by these women as liberation, a path to a place where the anxiety which gripped them as they awaited the medical biopsy result, doctor's verdict, or mammogram finding could not get to them. Their PM surgery, the removal of the breasts, let them breathe free again.

Here, three women describe their medical experiences leading up to their prophylactic mastectomy. Sonia said, "I always had a lot of lumps, tumors and bumps. Every single thing. So, the cancer was always somewhat of a pressure in my mind ... I had many biopsies and my breasts were all cut up." Janice's experience was that she, "went for a mammogram and they thought they saw something. It was like a scary thing. So, that gave me an extra push to do it, even though, it wasn't, thank God. But just the fear of the possibility." Fay said, "I thought, you know, I don't want to do this anymore ... I didn't want this [the possibility of cancer] hanging over me."

Women describe feeling that they were "running scared." The experience of worrying and being saved from the feared cancer diagnosis by a negative biopsy result or negative ultrasound finding was for many a crystallizing moment. Rose recalls, "I had a cyst in my breast and I remember being paralyzed with fear, thinking what if it had been. So at that point I decided I was going to get my breast removed." For Kate:

> [i]t was a long drawn-out affair after having several medical scares in terms of doctors telling me, "I feel a lump. We have to do some surgery." I had that happen twice. I think the last straw was when I went in for my usual every-six-months exam, and there was a yearly mammogram, and I had a discharge, which, completely, you know, again, here I am, the ticking time bomb. I just said, "I can't live like this anymore. I have to do something." That's what the doctor recommended [a PM].

Some women started having breast biopsies very early. Since young women tend to have denser breasts, it is often difficult to interpret their mammograms which may lead to, especially in families with significant family history of breast cancer, the recommendation that anything suspicious be biopsied. Valerie says, "I started, I think, when I was nineteen having biopsies. It was benign. I had lumps come and go. Then when I had my next biopsy, my tissues had started to change." Fay reported having had benign tumors removed from her breast surgically since she was 13. Her history illustrates the fact that it takes some women many years to consider the possibility of undergoing a PM before they make the decision, which is often precipitated by frustration at a series of evaluative biopsies or other investigations of suspicious breast findings. Valerie says that, "[y]ears later, after basically I had been through the problems I'd had for twenty years, because I was 33 at the time, I had yet another lump." It was removed but the doctor found "something odd" and she was referred to a specialist in Boston. He offered an array of options, including PM. Valerie chose a conservative path of close surveillance for the next three years.

But what happened was as those three years went on, I became more and more, you know, just feeling insecure about my physical health. I kept getting these lumps and they would remove them. But, I mean, it was so scary to me that basically there was a day where coming down for more tests and more mammograms and sonograms and all these things in Boston, I just basically, it was, like "I've had enough." I thought, you know, I don't want to do this anymore. Otherwise from this, I'm a very healthy person. I'm a very vibrant, busy person. I didn't want this hanging over me all the time.

Emily told us that:

[s]tarting way back when I was 28 years old, so that was 21 years ago, I started having lumps come. I had numerous needle biopsies and open biopsies. I'd go on a little ways and then I'd get another lump and then they'd biopsy. They always came back negative. About two years before I had the actual mastectomies, I had a lump biopsied, and it came back. They didn't say it was cancer, but they couldn't say it wasn't cancer. Once again, it came back and they didn't say that it was cancer, but they couldn't say for sure a hundred percent that it wasn't. After going round and round the loop with various doctors and everything, everybody came to the general consensus that just close observation would be the best thing to do at that point.

   Then two years later, I had in the very same area where the lump had been before that they had never been able to decide one way or the other, I had a lump come back. . . . I went and had that done and went through the whole rigmarole again, going round and round. "We can't say it is cancer. We can't say it isn't cancer." The oncologist that was overseeing my participation in the clinical trials recommended the prophylactic mastectomy to me at that time.

   At that point in my life, I was just older . . . Two years makes a difference in how you think of yourself, your concept of everything and at that point I just wanted to get rid of them [my breasts]. I didn't want to go through this every year or two . . . It was just too much of a roller coaster emotionally to every six or eight months or a year to have to go through that again. I just didn't want to do it anymore.

CHILDREN: NOT REPEATING THE PAST

One of the most commonly voiced primary motivations for under-going bilateral PM is to try to ensure that one will be available to bring up one's children. Often, among the women we interviewed, this was contrasted with their experience of the early loss of their mothers to breast cancer. They were motivated by the strong desire to spare their children the devastation of having a sick mother who eventually dies while they still very much need her care.

Alice told us that "I never would have had it without kids, never in a million years. I did it because of them. Yes, *the* reason." Meredith said, "[Having children] was everything to my decision. I'm way too vain. If I did not have kids, I would not have done this. I would have taken the odds." Grace's motivation was, "I didn't want to leave my children without a mom. I wanted to be there. I wanted to know I was going to live a long time and be there to watch them grow up." And Joyce said, "I felt as a parent, I had to do something. So if my body gets a little bit changed, so what? It's better than dying and it better to be the mother to my children and bring them up the way I feel fit. No, I'm glad I did what I did because I don't have to worry."

Not letting her children down was paramount to Laura.

I always felt that if I got cancer that I would somehow have let them [my children] down by not having the surgery. That I didn't do everything that I could, which is kind of odd, but I just felt like I had to for them. I grew up, part of my years, without a mom. It wasn't fun and I wasn't going to let that happen to them. I was going to do whatever it took, as crazy as that sounds. But I think that having kids puts you in that position. I don't know that I would have done this had I not had children. I don't know if I would have felt this strong sense of self-preservation.

The desire not to repeat the past, to have children whose mother accompanies them through childhood, to avoid the pain of early loss was, for these women, a primary motive, one worth considerable sacrifice. While we will consider later the issues for younger, single women who consider PM, the safety of a known partner and the impetus to "be there" for one's children made it considerably more likely in our study for PM to have been elected by married women who had young children. "And it was like, now I had to really think about what was the most important part of this, and that [children] was the most important part. So, therefore, if I ended up with nothing in the end, as far as reconstruction, it suddenly really didn't matter to me. The only thing that mattered to me was that I don't die before my children grow up" [Fay].

To some of these women, the decision to have a PM did not feel like a choice when they had children. "I couldn't have, well, I mean I could have done it for [husband' name], but you have to do it for your kids" [Beth]. Meredith, recognizing that there remains some risk of breast cancer even after PM, said, "But I mean even if I get it when they're [my children] in their twenties, that's still, they're grown up and they didn't grow up with it. They're on their own."

In considering what their decision might have been if they did not have children, Meredith said it did not make a difference to her, but the majority seemed to feel that children represented whatever swing there was in their decision. "If I hadn't had kids, you can't say for sure, but I think I would have taken my chances to see what cards were dealt me."

It is not clear how women with children who do not select this ultimate surgical step construe the decision differently or whether some feel guilt for opting to preserve their physical integrity at possible risk to their children's future well-being. But the vast majority of women in our study who had chosen PM were mothers and attributed much of the decision towards PM to their wish that their children grow up with a mother.

BREAST DISINVESTMENT

A number of women in our study spoke disparagingly about their natural breasts, those which they had had removed. It is not clear if this is a defensive, post-hoc way of minimizing the loss which PM occasions. In some cases, however, there was evidence from earlier surgery for breast reduction, etc. that the dislike of or lack of identification with their breasts had been a more long-standing feature. Some women spoke of how unimportant their breasts were to their sense of themselves. "I was always small-chested, so my chest was not a big part of, I mean, a lot of people I've run into don't even know what I had done—I never had reconstruction—they just think I'm small-chested which I was before." [Chantal] Other women diminish the impact of their PM on their own sexual enjoyment, "They [her breasts] were never a real source of pleasure to me in the first place," Kristen revealed. Ingrid said of her husband, "He wasn't a breast man anyway, so that wasn't a loss on his part or a major travesty." Others played down the notion that breasts are important to women, viewing the social emphasis on breasts in our culture as a solely male construction.

> I don't know how to explain it to you because it's funny. Breasts are an appendage, and men make such a big deal out of them. I think women are made to feel like they are just an object anyway. So to remove them and put something in there that looks just as good or almost as good is not a big deal. [Meredith]

One factor in this disinvestment has to do with the attitudes the women had towards their breasts as sources of fear and betrayal. A woman who was only 30 years old described her breasts as "bombs that were going to go off." Joyce explained her lack of attachment to her breasts in this way.

> The relationship I had with my old breasts was an acrimonious relationship. We weren't really fond of each other in the sense that I always had a feeling that they were going to really kill me some day. So I was never particularly attached to them, because from a very young age I had learned to be very suspicious of them. I did monthly breast self-examinations in which they were on one side and I was on the other side.

In our sample, it seemed that there were few women who spoke with much passion of the pleasures which their original breasts provided either to them or to their partners. This may be a function of the retrospective nature of our study. It may be that this is a critical variable which is difficult to gauge in medical discussions about PM, but which affects in good measure which of the women at risk are even willing to consider PM. Most oncologists and surgeons speak to patients about the medical rationale for PM and about reconstructive options; there is typically little or no discussion of the negative aspects or personal or relational losses such surgery entails. While it would also seem critical for couples to consider the impact of PM on their sexual foreplay and pleasure, this did not seem to have been discussed at length by many of the women in our sample even with spouses, a subject we will consider in more depth in later chapters.

CHAPTER 3

Making the Decision

How long it takes for a woman to come to a decision about prophylactic mastectomy (PM) varies widely, with some thinking about it for years and others springing into action after hearing about a cancer diagnosis of a close relative or friend. How does the decision actually get made? What role do medical professionals play in this decision? What advice is considered helpful and what is less so? And how do women making this decision perceive it? Does it feel like this is their decision to make or that others really made it for them?

PHYSICIAN RECOMMENDATION: A FACTOR IN DECISION MAKING

As quotes from the previous chapter illustrate, the timely suggestion from an influential and respected other—a doctor, mother, sister, or friend—that prophylactic mastectomy would be a good choice can also play a pivotal role in a woman's decision making. However, as these quotes also illustrate, there has to be synchrony between the woman's state of mind and the recommendation or thinking about PM can be put on the back burner for years, even decades. The women interviewed for this study had their prophylactic mastectomies before data was available on the success of this surgery and thus, relied very heavily upon their doctors' recommendations. Prior to the availability of data on the efficacy of prophylactic mastectomy, oncologists and breast surgeons were very hesitant to "recommend" PM to women. The concern was widespread that PM is a disfiguring surgery and that its use in women without a cancer diagnosis is difficult to support in an era when most initial treatment for at least early stage breast cancer is a lumpectomy, without removal of the breast.

There has been something of a sea change in the medical world, however, occasioned by the data from the Mayo Clinic and from the Netherlands[1, 2] which showed that there was at least a 90 percent risk reduction for breast cancer in high and moderate risk women who underwent PM. This has led many physicians and surgeons to be more forthright about the benefits of PM and to offer clear recommendations that that is the safest and best course medically. Still, doctors acknowledge that, at least in the United States, many high risk women do not choose PM[3] and that the decision about PM is a highly personal one. This decision takes into consideration many factors involving past, present, and future concerns and experiences.

THE POWER OF MEDICINE

Women in our study who had elected PM expressed a wide range of feelings about the power of modern medicine. Some felt that the medical system had let them down or that doctors had failed to find cancers in other family members which, in turn, influenced them to want to have a PM in order to reduce their reliance on imperfect screening procedures. Others clearly trusted their doctors implicitly and felt that their doctors had their best long-term interest in mind in recommending that they consider a PM. Still other women reported mixed experiences, at first mistrusting their doctors, then finding one who seemingly understood them and their needs and made them feel comfortable with the decision to undergo PM.

Joyce, a woman at high risk trying hard to comply with recommendations for annual mammograms and MRIs, felt that a series of mistakes, i.e., loss of her prior mammogram results and failure to do MRIs of both breasts, made her afraid of "falling through the cracks" through inadequate screening and thus, subsequently developing cancer. This hastened her decision for prophylactic surgery: "Hey, if I'm counting on early diagnosis here, this isn't going to happen. I'd already made my decision, but it was pretty clear to me at this point when I walked into the room that I was getting a confirmation that this is how you slip through the cracks. Even though you're at high risk and everybody's really trying hard to take care of you, it's really easy for a series of slipups to happen."

For other women, their implicit faith in their doctors figured heavily in their decision. Superlatives occurred frequently as women talked about "worshipping" or "loving" their doctor, having "total faith . . . just quick right from the beginning. [Kristen]" Another woman confessed, "I was just in a mode with Dr. X. and I really didn't care what anybody else thought. I mean people had their opinions, but I didn't care. I was going to do it."

THE DECISION IS THE WOMAN'S TO MAKE

Even more than for many other medical procedures, the elective nature of PM for women without cancer allowed many physicians to feel that they could legitimately provide information about PM to patients, but that the final decision had to be made by the woman. Valerie said of her medical providers, "They gave me all the options. It was pretty much up to me what I wanted to do. They gave me all the risk-benefit ratios. Actually, when I made my decision, they kind of went along with me." Janice said of her doctor, "He always left the decision up to me." Harriet similarly said of her physician, "She just gave me her opinions about what she'd seen and how accurate she thought mammography and other things were. She didn't make the decision. Obviously, the decision was ours."

Being the final decision maker in this healthcare issue was what many women wanted. When we asked women who had not had breast cancer who had the most influence on their decision to undergo PM, many replied, "Me." Having this final authority, however, can also be burdensome. Fay revealed that:

> [The doctors] kept saying, "Well, you know, we could recommend it, but then the fact is you might never have really needed it, but you might never really have gotten cancer. So, therefore, it may seem like—you know, and that's a huge thing to do in your life, to have this kind of surgery. So we don't want to be the ones to tell you. It's got to be your choice." So it was a very difficult time for me. It was an unclear time, because that's a huge decision to make, and what if I really didn't need it and what if I don't handle having had that surgery well, you know, and all of those questions.

The question "What would you do if it was your wife, or daughter, or sister?" was frequently mentioned as the way women who wanted more advice sought out their doctors' opinion. Honest answers to this question helped many women make their own decisions. Ingrid said that:

> I asked him [her doctor], plainly, what he would do. He said, "I would, honestly, have them both removed. Given what I've heard, I would have them both done." So I, more or less, had my mind made up that that's what I would do anyway, so that's where the decisions went along. I said, "Fine, go ahead." I stepped right up to that base right away, I did. Then I said, "While you're at it, you know, you could make them a little perkier?"

For some women, it was a matter of repeatedly asking for opinions, often of different doctors, until they found one whose opinion mirrored their own. As Joyce told us, "I guess what I was doing was I was presenting my family history to different physicians and then just sort of judging their reactions to it to try to get an assessment of my level of risk." In some cases, it was the opposite tactic, with the doctor broaching the subject of PM repeatedly over time, until a point where the woman was ready to think seriously about this surgical option.

Women felt that it was "respectful" of doctors to clearly see the decision as one which the patient ultimately was in charge of. This decision often occurred after considerable discussion, when trust had developed between the two. Kate said, "When she [the surgeon] came right out and offered the prophylactic mastectomy, I felt like here is a person who—I felt very close to her. Her mom had gone through it, and she was a woman. So I didn't feel like this was some sort of surgeon's answer to anything. I didn't feel that way about it, that she was just too quick to put me under the knife." Sometimes the trust and perception of empathetic response occurred more quickly when empathy was present. "I think she was absolutely incredible. She was there for me, and the empathy was genuine. I still feel very comfortable with her, and I just met her prior to that. [Laura]"

Both male and female surgeons were generally seen as empathetic and caring. Little acts of kindness, such as a call shortly before surgery to check on how the woman was feeling in anticipation of the procedure or finding a pink rose next to her bed, placed there by her surgeon, when she woke up from surgery meant a great deal to these women. Not all experiences, however, were positive. Harriet told us that "[t]he truth is we did go to some doctors that were very against it. There were a few doctors that were very strongly against it. One doctor said to me, 'It's a deforming operation, really. You shouldn't do it.' But, in general, I felt very comfortable with the doctor I had. It felt like we had very good communication." Only one woman complained that male doctors she went to "thought I was crazy," which she attributed to being "because men think women are supposed to have breasts. [Kristen]"

Some women felt that a mother, sister, or brother were important in their decision making, sometimes because of the advice they offered, but sometimes because of issues related to the multigenerational breast cancer risk. Valerie said her mother had the most influence on her decision.

> Not that she encouraged it at all. She kind of left it up to me, whatever I wanted to do. But just that I figured not only did she go through it and come out okay, and I probably could do the same. But I didn't want to take any risks and possibly not be around for her. I still had—it was still fresh in my mind that she was still having bone scans every year; that possibly it [cancer] could show up in her. She really needed, I thought, to have me around; me, the only nurse in the family. I resigned myself to the fact that that was my lot in life, taking care of my parents if they become ill.

INFLUENCE OF FAMILY MEMBERS: SPOUSES AND SIGNIFICANT OTHERS

Besides the woman herself, her sexual partner may be presumed to be the person most immediately affected by a woman's decision to have her breasts surgically removed. Classically, attention has been slow to come to the sexual and relationship ramifications of mastectomy. Many men have reported anxiety about whether or how to talk with their wives about feelings they might have about the loss of her breasts. Husbands and sexual partners are often given little room for their thoughts or feelings to be considered—other than appreciation for pure statements of support for the woman's decision. While most women reported discussing their decision with their husband or partner, quite a few women, especially those without cancer, voiced very strong feelings that this was only their decision. It was almost as if any discussion of mixed emotions about the decision was heresy, even though the woman herself might have such ambivalence. Kristen said "I was going to do it, no matter what anybody thought, and if I had a husband that was going to walk because I got my breasts taken off, then adios." Irene felt that she "probably would have had it regardless [of whether or not husband supported her] because I was so convinced it was the right thing. But it certainly made it much easier for me to make that decision and feel good about that decision by having his support." Vicky simply said "I came home and told my husband, 'I'm doing it.' There were no questions." Her husband, she says, is:

> pretty laid back and he's not too medically knowledgeable. He knows me well enough that he kind of knows that if I've made up my mind to do something, that I'll probably do it no matter what he thinks. But he wasn't openly against it or openly for it. He was just kind of there, neutral. Just very much typically like he is about anything.

Clearly, support from husbands was very important, sometimes pivotal. Harriet said, "My husband and I just came to the decision together . . . I mean, he wanted me to do it also. I don't think I would have done it if he had not wanted to." And Laura reported, "The entire time he was extremely supportive, always there. I don't think I could have gone through the whole—I'm not sure I would have done it, to tell you the truth, if I didn't have a good relationship with him, because I think I did it for us."

Few women acknowledged how challenging a role this was for their husband. Beth said, "I don't think he always knew what to say to make it easier, but I think he held my hand and told me it would be okay and we would be all right."

Interestingly, it was rare to hear empathy for the implications of the woman's decision for her spouse, but there were a few such statements. Kate said, "I mean, he was obviously going to let this be my decision . . . My husband was very, very positive. It was almost like I told him I was going to go in and have my hair cut. I didn't feel that he was going to mourn the loss of anything. That was just how he made me feel. But he definitely left it up to me. He didn't express any kind of questioning or whatever or challenge me or ask me to wait or anything like that. He has known the anxiety I have felt over the years."

Alice mused about the impact of her decision to have a PM on her husband:

> You know, I did something pretty big that impacted my husband and me a lot. Even though he never complains ever, it's still, I feel kind of bad for him. You know, I had to do this and—I mean, he's

been great, but I know that I've done something that maybe wasn't necessary and look, the society that we live in . . . He's given up a lot and I feel bad . . . . [When *Victoria Secrets* are on TV] I feel bad for him. I do. I feel bad. You know, he's great. He is. But I feel like, "Poor guy."

Not a Breast Man

A remarkable number of women referred to their partners as "not a breast man." This phrase was offered as an explanation for why their decision about prophylactic mastectomy was not difficult for their partners or husbands. "In really plain English, he wasn't a breast man anyway, so that wasn't a loss on his part or a major travesty." [Ingrid] "He's not a breast man anyway, is how I explain it. That's not what he concentrates on." [Meredith] Julia reported that her husband told her, "'I just want you here for the next 50 years. It doesn't matter to me,' he said. 'Obviously, I'm not a breast man.'"

There seemed some similarity between the breast disinvestment statements of some women and their assessments of the lack of importance of their breasts to their husbands. These views seemed to make women feel better about their decision, less like they were taking something important away from themselves or their partners. It also seemed to imply that there were no feelings of ambivalence or loss which the women themselves experienced. These are, of course, the women's assessments of the relative lack of importance of breasts to their partner's sexual interest. These are women who have not had cancer; cancer has not altered their breasts or been a source of medical intervention, except, possibly, for biopsies. However, some high risk women focused considerable worry on their breasts and this may have contributed to a lack of sexual pleasure involving the breasts for both men and women in some couples. Data is not available on how these men, if speaking freely, would have described their reactions. We might surmise a greater complexity if the men were interviewed, though, without doubt, the overwhelming concern would be about the woman's longevity and freedom from cancer.

Single Ladies

Not every woman was lucky enough to have a supportive spouse or to have her decision making occur during a calm period in her marriage. Valerie and her husband were "having a lot of issues" over the nine to twelve months during which she made her decision about PM. She says that her health became her focus, not her deteriorating marriage. Valerie found her husband not to be helpful. She was embarrassed when he joked in front of a surgeon about what kind of implants she could get after the surgery which, she said, "reinforced where my priorities actually were." She and her husband had joined a couples group a few months before her surgery. The night before the surgery, after not having talked about the surgery at all in the couples group, she finally brought it up and "broke down completely," something she had not experienced before anywhere. Valerie says she knew that things with her husband would change, one way or the other, after the surgery. While she hoped their relationship might improve, that was not what occurred. After the surgery, she felt that he was even less supportive and her anger at him increased. She says they realized they were not compatible and subsequently, they divorced.

Meredith was aware before she married her husband that she wanted to have a PM.

> We got married when I was 26. I told him before I married him that I was going to do it someday, so he married me knowing that ... He's a nice guy and a smart guy. He said, "Pretty much whatever you want to do, you know." His mother died of melanoma and his sister had some weird thing, multimyeloma or something like that and so he has got a lot of cancer in his family and so he knows that the risk is real, you know.

Advice: If the Husband Does not Understand

Janice had advice for women whose husbands initially were not in agreement about their PM decision:

> Sit down with your husband, talk it over, go out to dinner, talk with him without the kids around, without any environment around. Just sit and talk and have a quiet moment and ask him how he would really feel about it. Take that aspect of it and then go sit. If your husband still felt, "No, you shouldn't have it done because I think you're less of a woman or something," then maybe what you need to do is just to bring in a physician friend just to try to explain it to him. Have him come to the next doctor's visit with you, just sit and talk and listen to his aspect,

because you've got a lot more thoughts in your mind how you see it, but the surgeon can kind of help him understand it a little bit better because you're seeing it through a different angle than what he is. Sometimes just bringing someone else in that he knows you've seen for a long time, that kind of helps it.

Sandra summary statement was, "I think anybody considering this [PM surgery] has to realize that it's going to have a tremendous impact. I think a good relationship can withstand it and one that has problems or a relationship where you're not used to working through difficulties of this sort, it's going to be challenging. There is no doubt about it."

CHILDREN

Having prophylactic surgery causes sufficient day-to-day disruption in family routines that a mother, even of young children, feels that she owes her children an explanation about why she is having surgery and what she is having done. This may mean that discussions about high familial cancer risk may come up sooner than would otherwise have been the case, although, not necessarily full discussions about such risk or all about surgery and reconstruction. Depending on family communication style and the age of the children, children may have things to say about PM which their mothers take into consideration in their decision making.

Alice at 50 had children old enough to remember their grand-mother's and aunt's breast cancers:

They remembered that, you know, I went through it when my sister was sick and I was always talking about it. Then I said I want to do something so that I don't get breast cancer. I remember my son, saying, "Well, what can you do?" I said, "Take them off." He looked at me like I was kidding, like, are you crazy? "What?" I said, "Yes, but there is an operation where I can take them off so that maybe I won't get cancer in them if they're not there. So then I can have some kind of operations to put something back so that it looks . . . " Then I explained it to them. Then, pretty much after that time, I didn't talk about it for years. There was really not much to say. They'd known I would do it and they didn't bring it up and I didn't bring it up.

"My family was wonderful," Julia said. They told her:

"Go for it [the PM surgery]. Just go for it." My girls would joke
with me. They are both like C/D cups. They look at me and they
go, "Mom, nobody's going to [be able to] tell." So, there was tons
of humor about it in our family. They said, "Whatever you want."
I told them what every doctor said. They said, "I don't think your
decision should be hard at all." . . . I explained it to my kids is that,
"I'm taking a more aggressive route but I want you to learn that it
can be managed if you're aggressive." I said, "I'm never going to
let it beat me."

Vicky also strongly conveyed the hope that knowledge of her PM
experience would help her daughters be aggressive in their breast
management.

I informed my daughters on it and told them to be very aggressive
on theirs. . . . I talked to them that I was going to have this
because I didn't want to get cancer, because I've had enough—
nothing was ever showing up as precancerous, even with the cysts
that they removed and whatever. But I just thought I was running
on a different track, that I was just trying to run ahead of it and I
wasn't going to do that. It was a decision I just felt that I needed
to do rather than go another year and say, "Oh, there's another
cyst and there's another one." Why risk tumors and all that stuff,
I didn't want to go there . . . They just accepted it. They have
been well versed on all of that, with their grandmother and everything, that they just didn't. They accepted it with no I just told
them that the biggest thing is for them to be aggressive themselves, because high risk tumors are in the family. Just to keep a
heads-up on all of that.

Some children are too young to understand the full maternal
message and warnings about breast cancer. With young children,
finding age-appropriate ways to talk with them may be challenging.
Rose took a very creative approach to talking to her three- and five-
year-old children at the time of her surgery. "What I told my kids
was that it was like a stuffed animal. What they were going to do is
they're taking out my old stuffing and putting in new stuffing."
One of the concerns mothers have in telling children about PM is
who will the children talk to about it and whether the woman can

maintain the level of privacy she is comfortable with about her surgery. It may not always be the children who reveal their mother's plans; they may be affected by the way other children talk about their mother's surgery. Some of the discussion may reflect the sense of amazement (and possible underlying discomfort) which was apparent in the response of Fay's daughter. Further discussion and the child's observation of the mother's level of comfort about the surgery may allay his or her fears and reduce his or her sense that this is a strange thing to do.

Fay says,

When you talk to children, like their friends like the word "boobs," and all that makes little kids giggle and all, and my daughter had experienced one moment that somebody in our town, because it's a small town—had gotten wind of what I was doing and some parent said something in front of their child. The child was in her class and it was a boy. I remember he said something to her while I was at the hospital about, you know, he announced this in class, "My mom says your mom is doing something to her boobies" and all the kids kind of laughed. It wasn't a real big deal. But that was probably a reason for me to be a little careful about how much I said publicly. But there was nobody I tried avoiding telling it. I was very fine with the decision and I'm not ashamed or embarrassed or anything.

SISTERS

The relationship between sisters is one of the most intensely affected by recognition of the hereditary or familial predisposition to breast cancer and the decision about PM. When one sister seriously considers PM, there is often pressure, direct or indirect, on other similarly-aged sisters to also consider the decision to have this surgery. In families where genetic testing has been done, sisters who had tested negative for the familial mutation would be exempted from such consideration, but those who had not been tested, who tested positive, or had indeterminate results would likely be encouraged by their doctors and, at least in many cases, by their sisters or other relatives to also think about having a PM. This mirror effect—if this recommendation for PM applies to me now, it must also apply to my sisters—brings some sisters closer together. It can be a great comfort to have someone

who knows the family history, and may know or even share the doctors involved with whom one can talk about not only the personal
impact of PM, and also about the expected impact on other family
members. Sisters not infrequently come to medical appointments
together for genetic counseling or testing or for pre-surgery talks with
surgeons, since information that applies to one may apply to both.
(However, since surgical and reconstructive decisions involve body
shape, size, and medical history, there may be limits to the degree that
such advice applies to both sisters.) While the timing may vary
depending on age and circumstance, there are families in which sisters
all choose to undergo PM.

There are, however, families in which sisters are not perceived as
close allies in this process, but, instead the decision around PM leads
to discussions between family members in which emotions are heightened, anger is aroused, and differences are silhouetted. Rather than
having similarities or even respectful disagreements triumph, fear
seems to be a significant underlying cause when sisters find little support from each other. One woman's decision to undergo PM arouses
fear in the sisters which, often unexpressed, leads some to distance
themselves from the sister considering surgery and from thinking personally about cancer risk and what they feel are extreme, risk-reducing
options. Any revisiting of the cancer risk in the family brings up fear-
inducing memories of previous illnesses and deaths of family members
from breast cancer. Unresolved anger may surface about who did or
did not care for a mother during her bout with cancer, how a mother's
cancer was discovered (or not) and treated, and circumstances around
the mother's death and burial.

Jealousy is not infrequently heard in discussions about hereditary
breast cancer. Older generations envy the fact that the younger generations have more options; younger generations envy the fact that the
older ones did not have to worry about hereditary cancer, genetic testing, and prophylactic surgery until they were much older. Sisters may
envy each other for where they are in their lives when consideration of
PM is recommended to them. An older sister may envy her younger
sister for having more time to consider the option of surgery. A younger sister may envy her older married sister with children because she
is at a more stable point in her life and already has a supportive partner. Feelings between sisters may become particularly brittle, due to
the mirroring impact of the information.

My sister, actually she lives in Boston. She was supportive, but it also scared her that this, I mean, to actually have it done ... Well, the only one I would discuss it with would be my sister, and she has somewhat of a denial attitude, and her breasts are very important to her. They're important to her husband. She would never have that done. She's just in kind of denial and just wants to take her chances, which to me is a little foolish, but she does get herself regular checks ... There was times when she couldn't be there for me because she was so scared [Kristen].

No. I mentioned it [genetic testing], and they [my sisters] said, "Oh, hogwash," basically. They don't want to know just—they just don't think it's a possibility, I think. Because one sister did have a mass that was benign. The other sister just won't even bother going for mammograms. She totally has her head in the sand about this. I guess sometimes I get frustrated and other times I just have to resign myself to the fact that they are adults, and they're going to have to make their own decisions about things like that. [Valerie]

Some women were very disappointed by their sisters' reactions. Julia told us, "I have to say I did not get support from my sisters at all. At all, which was hurtful. I think it's because they're afraid. They just don't want to go there with me. They said, 'Well, I think you're a little overzealous.'"

Joyce said told us that:

I didn't speak to my sister about it [having a PM]. I just went ahead and did it ... My own sister has never even been for a mammogram. She can't talk about it. My family has had a very, very diverse reaction to my surgery ... No, no, I have never spoken to my sister about my experience. She's never asked me. We went to my cousin's funeral in May. My cousin was buried because of breast cancer. The gene result had not come in. My sister, as that time, knew that I'd had a prophylactic mastectomy, and she completely avoided the whole subject. She can't talk to me about it. Yet, she's at the same level of risk as I was, and she sat on my mother's bed and was told that she should have a prophylactic mastectomy. So she has had the identical experience I have had, other than where my experience parted from hers coming to Boston. ... But the fact that at the time I was seeing Dr. X. in Boston, I went to my sister, and I had to speak to her about the cousin on my father's side of the family that Dr. X. wanted to have tested. At that time, she said, "Why are you doing this?" I said, "Because I'm looking into the possibility of a prophylactic mastectomy," and she just completely flipped out and the conversation ended right there. In light of that conversation, she told me that she had never had a mammogram, and she was forty-five when that conversation occurred.

Hanna felt it was hard to find grounds for common understanding with her sister about her decision to have a PM:

I have a sister that I've talked with about it. She said she would do it if her doctor says for her to do it. Right now, they've got her, the doctor that she's seeing over at [X] Hospital thinks that I shouldn't have done it. Really, I have a hard time to want to get into topics with people on it, unless they are going through it, because people—I don't know. It's hard when you have a family member say, "Why did you do such a thing?" They just don't quite understand where I'm at or where I was at or where I'm at today.

Support from sisters can be particularly meaningful at this time because of the resonance in their circumstances and the knowledge that to be supportive, a sister may have overcome her own worries for herself as well as for her sister. Support from a sister with breast cancer may feel especially important because of its selfless concern, a wish for the still-healthy sister to avoid the trials of the ill sister.

Probably my sister who was [the most influential person]—well, both my sisters, the one who diagnosed and my youngest sister who is actually an OB/GYN. And then my husband. My sister who was diagnosed with the cancer said, "You know, it's time. We know what we're up against now." She said to both myself and my youngest sister, "You guys should have the surgery.... [Irene]

She [my younger sister] was here with me through the whole surgery. She was watching my son. She was here from start to finish ... My sister, who's two years younger than me, the following year she went to her doctor, who she has the same fibrous tumors that I had, and her doctor opted to do the same thing. She had her bilateral mastectomy as well. Two other sisters opted not to ... They [my other sisters] just were aggressive enough doing the mammograms that they felt that they didn't want to go that route. [Vicky]

OTHER RELATIVES

Some women find their families to be uniformly positive about their decision to have a PM. Ingrid said, "Well, I had the complete approval of my entire family in doing it. I think with them they knew what would probably be in store for me. There wasn't any second thoughts. There really wasn't." Laura told us broadly that "[m]y extended family has been wonderful."

The opinions of male relatives (fathers, brothers, etc.) tend to have less influence, although in rare cases, male relatives (beyond husbands and sons) played important roles in decision making. One woman credited her brother, a doctor, with having helped her by gathering medical information and discussing the issues with her as she made up her mind.

Not all family members were initially supportive, although, with time, some came to be. Alice said that,

> [m]y dad kind of thought I shouldn't [have the surgery], but he didn't push. He just [said] "What if?" He thought, "Just don't mess with it, you know. It's pretty drastic. Don't mess with it." So I didn't really heed that, but I respected him telling me what he thought, and I still think about that . . . They [my cousins] thought we were sort of—they just weren't crazy about the idea. They didn't want to know. But I think now that they've had kids and both of them are married, they're changing their mindsets, so they're all starting to go through the procedures [gene testing].

Meredith's brothers were divided in their opinions:

> It's funny, because my family—well, my brother Steven was pretty supportive. But my brother Al was actually angry about me doing it. He thought I was mutilating myself and it was unnecessary or it wouldn't work anyway. Then, like a month before I was hooked up for surgery, stuff came out about Tamoxifen, and I actually called my mother's old doctor, who remembered all those years later. He said it was called positively charged, it was hormone driven, just the same as he had told me, and that Tamoxifen might not work that well anyway. So, my brothers were calling me, going, "You don't have to do this. They have Tamoxifen now." I'm like, "It's not that simple, you know" . . . I never really quite understood. I think he just was horrified.

Irene faced opposition as well from her family:

> I think, certainly, I had some family members, even on my husband's side of the family, who initially thought, "Is she nuts? She's going to go get her breasts cut off." But, I think once I talked to them and they understood the full extent of the situation, I mean they were aware of my family history, and then once they became aware of the genetic situation, I think everyone once they understood the full situation and what the real risks were, everyone realized that this was a good thing. It makes a lot of sense.

PRIVACY

Who a woman tells about her prophylactic mastectomy may depend on the family relationships, other ongoing matters of concern, and also on the woman's views about privacy. Some women were quite open among relatives and friends. Other women, either initially or permanently, decide not to talk about PM with many people. Some women were worried that, if people knew about the surgery, they would reduce them to their breasts, looking at their chest area, not at their eyes, when they spoke to them. Others worried that talking to too many people might elicit too many unwanted opinions that might cause a woman to waiver in her decision to have surgery:

> I very purposefully did not speak to any other members of my family, because I didn't want anybody to shake my resolve. I had made this decision and I didn't want to hear anything negative and I was very conscious of that. My brother came to take care of me, as did my best friend come to take care of me after the surgery and to see me through. I had the surgery in September. In November, I picked up the telephone and I phoned the only woman in my mother's generation who had survived breast cancer, as sort of the representative of my mother's generation. I called her up and I told her. I asked her to, my words were "Could you just sort of let it out on the grapevine? I don't want it to cause too much. Don't make a big pronouncement about it, just as you would speak to people when you see them" . . . She let it drop like an atomic bomb.
>
> Two days later, I got a very serious phone call from a cousin of mine who said "So, you decided to do this? Tell me, why did you

decide to do this?" . . . What I've learned about this experience from my own family is, is that my own family's reaction to it is extremely diverse. Even the one physician in my family, a female physician, she can't talk about it. To me, that was really interesting when a physician doesn't want to hear much about it. [Joyce]

Other women in our study felt similarly about privacy issues and their decision to have a PM:

Let me put it to you this way. I'm a very private person. What goes on with my life is nobody else's business. Other than that, my immediate family, being my brother and sister, and close friends, they knew all about it. People that I worked with or anything like that, it's none of their business. [Sonia]

You know what, I'm a pretty private person. I didn't tell any of my friends beforehand to get any kind of feedback. Also, because, if you've gone through a death in your family, you know that people look at you in a different way, you can feel that. Unless you know of somebody who has gone through a similar thing with you, it's a tremendous thing to lay on somebody else I have found in my life, having lost two parents and a sister. It's a big thing to lay on somebody who maybe hasn't gone through that in their life. They can't possibly understand. So I am more comfortable not discussing those things. Unless someone else has gone through that, then I know they can relate to that kind of thing. So I'm pretty private that way. [Kate]

Sandra worried about burdening people and felt it might be giving them too much information about herself, especially after they knew about her sister's recent illness:

I didn't tell a lot of people. I mean I told close friends, and, of course, my family knew. But I didn't advertise it because I thought, you know, it's an unusual surgery to have. There was a quality of when my sister was very sick, I really felt like we were going through stuff that made me feel that I was sort of outside the normal realm of life . . . I didn't want to sort of continue with that. I didn't want to say, "Hi, acquaintances from work, you just saw me go through this terrible ordeal with my sister, and now I'm going to do this. I'm just continuing this stuff that's so much outside the realm of everyday life of our society." So, I didn't want that, and I was really conscious of that.

A few women felt their openness about their decision to have this surgery was not rewarded. Julia felt "terrible opposition from my friends and my peers" and Fay felt misunderstood. Those people she did tell seemed unable to believe she had not been diagnosed with cancer:

> The public opinion is you would never—"Why would anybody do something like that if they didn't have to? If she did it, even though I could swear I heard her say she never had cancer, she must have had cancer." Because I've had so many people say to me throughout the years things, to the effect, "So your health, you're really okay now?"
>
> I said, "I was fine before; I'm more fine now."
>
> But the people—or they'll even say like "So is the cancer like all taken care of?"
>
> I said, "I never had cancer," and they have a real hard time hearing it, and understanding it, because I've explained it very clearly to people, and had those same people come back at me and say, "Oh, I'm so glad you're well now."
>
> I said, "I was well then."

Sonia had, "lots of people telling me, you know, 'My God, without your breasts, you lost your femininity.' It's like, 'No, I haven't.' My femininity was never in my breasts. It was more on my brain, and what I have to contribute."

CHAPTER 4

Preparing for Surgery: Practically, Physically, and Emotionally

TRUST IN SURGEONS

Some women knew their surgeons from prior surgical experiences—childbirth or breast reduction—and some met them for the express purpose of discussing prophylactic mastectomy (PM). Many women met with several surgeons, a few with many, before making their decision. Most women wanted to know from the surgeon, Did the doctor believe that PM was an appropriate surgery for her? The question they had to answer for themselves was, Do I feel comfortable enough with this surgeon to schedule the surgery? Because this surgery was not universally endorsed, especially for women who sought PM before the publication of the landmark studies showing over 90 percent breast cancer risk-reduction, there was much relief when women found a surgeon who shared their belief that this was a legitimate and, often, an important method of reducing risk. A few women felt if they had not found a surgeon willing to endorse PM, they would not have undergone the surgery. Others felt that they would simply have continued to interview surgeons until they found one who did favor PM for them. In many ways, it seemed that women were seeking approval, not only for the surgery, but also for their reasoning skills and abilities. They, after all, often had started on the road to find a surgeon, against the advice of family and friends. Not all women found the comfort they wanted, but for those who did, their appreciation was great. The congruence and approval they felt when they found a surgeon whose views coincided with their own seemed to extend to personal approval, which may have contributed to the extent of the praise for many of the surgeons. And when the surgeon was also personally supportive, women were ecstatic.

Interviewing surgeons and plastic surgeons until the right match was found was a common theme among the women in our study:

> I had talked to the plastic surgeon about the pros and the cons of the prophylactic mastectomy, what it was going to mean to my quality of life.... I have to tell you I'm a really fussy person. I went to several plastic surgeons. You can imagine, what the heck, I work in a medical school. I don't like that one, didn't like that one, didn't like that. But I was going for opinions everywhere I could find them, and I'm fortunate enough that I have the kinds of connections that I needed. [Joyce]

> I interviewed many plastic surgeons. A bit complicated, because you have to have, when you pick a plastic surgeon, you have to be aware that they have to have privileges to do surgery wherever your surgeon is. So that was kind of hard to hear, but you need to really interview many of the plastic surgeons. [Rose]

> The truth is we did go to some doctors that were very against it. There were a few doctors that were very strongly against it. One doctor said to me, "It's a deforming operation, really. You shouldn't do it." But, in general, I felt very comfortable with the doctor I had. It felt like we had very good communication. [Harriet]

> I first saw a different doctor, a surgeon, and she totally turned me off... I'd never go back and see her, and I think that's something important. You have to feel good with the person who's doing it. If there's any uncomfortable—if you're uncomfortable, find someone else.... She was very cold. She was very—did not take into consideration my feelings, what I was feeling. I don't know if I just caught her on a bad day... Someone that you feel comfortable with is very important. If there's any bit of uneasiness, don't do it with them. Find someone else. [Chantal]

Praise was high when a woman found a doctor whom she saw eye to eye with. Beth said that "Dr. X was probably the best thing that ever walked the face of this earth for me... As he said, 'You've got more of a chance of getting hit by a bus than you getting breast cancer' ... I'm one of the ones that had the support that was there." Kristen similarly idealized her doctors:

> I have all the faith in the world in Dr. X. She's a wonderful surgeon, wonderful human being. She's sincere as a physician. I don't know. I guess I've seen a lot of physicians in my life, and to me, she's the most dedicated. She really cares about her patients as a person. So I would say Dr. X and Dr. Y. They were both very knowledgeable doctors, and they made me comfortable in what I had decided ... The insurance drove me nuts, but then it was all straightened out because of Dr. X., the saint that she is. I had total faith in her, it just clicked right from the beginning .... I think that I was just in a mode with Dr. X, and I really didn't care what anybody else thought .... Yes, I mean, we were compatible from the beginning, and she was so honest and forthright with me that, you know, I felt totally comfortable with her. To be honest with you, I don't know if I ever would have had the surgery done if I hadn't had her for a surgeon.

Sandra's doctors filled her with respect for her own decision making:

> I felt that as a team they would be able to preserve my life and, in many ways, sort of preserve my body. Even if they hadn't been, I think quite honestly, I think even if plastic surgery was not available, I would have gone through with it ... They were great [my doctors]. They said it was sort of an extreme measure to take. I mean they were very clear that this was not something that I had to do. But they were also clear in letting me know that this was an option for me and that this was something I might want to consider. I think they were really respectful. Every doctor I worked with was very respectful about it. I think if I had decided not to do it, nobody would have judged me harshly. But they were supportive when I did make the decision, and I think it was obvious how clear I was on it.

Me Going to a Plastic Surgeon?

Many of the women who have had plastic surgery in the context of PM remember that they were somewhat shocked at the idea they were going to see a plastic surgeon. Plastic surgery, in their minds, was associated with cosmetic procedures such as breast enhancement, tummy tucks, or face lifts.

> I was in his office and there's all these rich women complaining about who gives better collagen injections for lips. "There's one in New York that does your veins good", and I'm thinking, "Oh, my God, what am I doing?" But maybe he was happy to do something normal. I don't know. But he had done a lot of reconstruction, and even he was very supportive . . . I don't think I could have done it if I didn't think they had reconstruction. [Kate]

TALKED INTO IT?

Some women felt they had benefitted from quite strong, direct advice from their doctors. One woman who had previously had very large breasts—"almost an E cup" and had previous breast reduction down to a C cup, originally thought when she was considering PM, she would entirely forego reconstruction. Her surgeon felt this was not a good psychological decision and told her so, though he did leave the final decision to her.

> The reason I was talked into it [having a reconstruction], I am a C, D . . . he said, "You really don't want to go flat-chested. You really want to have something, because it will be that traumatic." I said, "I'm just going to be a tee-shirt woman." But he said you really should [have reconstruction], and I think he probably was correct, because he's been there more than I have. I don't regret having it, but he kind of said, "You really don't want to go from where you were to nothing. It will be traumatic." I thought he was wonderful, so I agreed with him. He wasn't talking me into it per se, but he did give me the right answer. [Vicky]

Visuals: Seeing Photographs and Drawings

Women were very grateful to be able to see photographs and drawings of the surgery and reconstruction of other women when offered by surgeons or nurses. This enabled many to come to a better understanding of what to expect from their own surgery and reconstruction.

> That was really the cosmetic surgeon. He was so positive for it and in looking at my body and saying, "Well, of course, I can

do a wonderful job, something that is going to make you just feel that much better about all this." Then he showed me pictures, and he said, "You're going to be under surgery anyway. You're not unhealthy. You don't have cancer. There's no reason for it." I guess I asked all the usual questions, because of breast implants these days have come under such scrutiny and things like that. We talked about saline versus other things and that kind of thing. He was instrumental. [Kate]

Dr. X was very good every time I went there. She's very straightforward, and she did a lot of drawings. She would sit across the desk from me with a paper and pencil and draw pictures for me . . . . In fact, it was more helpful to me than some of the things that she tried to explain to me verbally. If I didn't get it, she'd draw me a picture. [Kristen]

ESTABLISH WHERE THE INCISIONS WILL BE

Valerie recounted that she had had a near terrible surgical PM experience. She had talked to other women who had undergone PM, all of whom had told her that the incision lines would be beneath her breasts. On the day of the surgery, however, her surgeon told her he was planning to put her suture lines on top of her breasts. "He made these lines on top of my breasts. He says, 'We're going to make the incisions here and here . . . ' So I thought to myself, 'Oh, my goodness, I haven't said that—.' I mean, I was on the stretcher my—I was in my gown and my hair was all under the cap and everything . . . Good thing I established that before I went in. That would have been a horrible thing."

PRACTICAL PREPARATIONS

Having made the decision for PM, a woman must prepare herself and her family for the event of the surgery itself. This involves deciding when it will take place, which can, by its very elective nature, be somewhat difficult. This year? Which month? When the kids are in school or out of school? Near the holidays or avoid the holidays? When work can spare me? Another concern to consider may be when the spouse or partner can get time off from work to be with his wife in the hospital, with the children, or both. Then, there are considerations of when the surgeon is available and when he or she can coordinate his or her schedule with that of the plastic surgeon, if one is also involved. In families with young children, there should be planning for who will fill in for the mother's tasks, such as taking children to and from school and activities, making meals, being present at sports events, etc. This may involve having a grandparent travel from another city or another part of the country, which adds another layer of planning and preparation.

Whether one involves friends and neighbors depends on how widely the woman wants to disseminate the news of her surgery. Each step may involve an explanation of what is being done and why and why now, if such conversations with these individuals have not been ongoing. This process can itself be tiring and feel invasive. And while much of this would be the same if the surgery were medically necessary, the fact of its electiveness may increase the burden of explanation for the woman.

TALKING WITH CHILDREN

Preparing for PM surgery also marks a point at which children need to be provided with explanations and an opportunity to ask their questions about what is happening to their mother. Especially if the children are of early elementary school age, they may not have been included in family discussions about the prospect of surgery or recent doctor visits. The news that their mother is about to have surgery may come as a shock to them. They need a true explanation of what kind of surgery their mother will undergo and some reasons why she is having this surgery. Children this age quickly move the focus of concern to themselves, i.e., what does this mean for me? Their questions can be at a very mundane level, "Who will pick me up from school on Monday?" or, especially with slightly older daughters, "Will I have to have this surgery when I grow up?" Making sure that after telling the child about the surgery, a parent asks them what they are thinking or worrying about is very important in order to know at which level to offer reassurance. Unfortunately, it is impossible to guess all of the things a child could possibly connect to their ideas of a mother having surgery and returning home without her breasts or with much-changed breasts.

How one explains prophylactic mastectomy to children of different ages depends heavily on:

- the style of communication that is typical for the family,
- the family experience with breast cancer,

- the particular emotional qualities of the child and their needs for security, and
- the comfort of the parents with their decision.

If the children are aware that there have been family members with breast cancer, the discussion would be likely to start there. A possible discussion might go like this:

As you know, Grandma and Aunt Sue both had breast cancer. I really want to do everything I can to make sure I don't get breast cancer. While I can't be absolutely sure, the best thing I can do is to have some surgery to take off my breasts. I don't need my breasts now for feeding you, like I did when you were babies. So I can have the surgery and not worry about breast cancer. It will mean I will have to be in the hospital for _____ [however long it will be)].

When I come home, I may not feel well for a couple of days and I will have to rest and sleep a lot. I won't be able to pick up _____ [toddler's name]. I may want to stay in bed and have my meals there like you do when you are not feeling well. I will ask you to be a little quieter than usual and probably not have friends over for a few days. It will be better for you to have play dates at your friends' houses for those days. You can help Daddy bring me breakfast and dinner and I would really like it if you wanted to watch a movie or a TV show with me.

In about a week, I will feel better and be up and around, but I may still not be able to drive you to school or pick you up because I will have stitches and still have to heal more. But Grandma or other relative is coming to stay with us when I am in the hospital and she will drive you to school or to your friends' houses for play dates. I will be able to be home for about a month from work, so we will get to spend some more time together during the week, which will be fun, especially as I feel better. Now, can you tell me what questions you have about all this?

This could be modified by any real-life experience the child has had related to surgery or cancer. You will want to reassure him or her that you do NOT HAVE cancer and that you will not die from this surgery. When Irene was asked how would she talk to her (still very young) children about surgery, she replied:

Well, I think, for us, it would probably come up in the context of our family history and how my mother died and how my sister was diagnosed and my sister did die from her cancer. So, I think it will probably come up in the context of that, because we spend a lot of time with my sister's son. So, he spends a lot of time with us now since my sister died. I think in kind of the process of talking through what happened to my sister and all of that, I think it would probably come up in that context, because I'm sure at some point they will have the fear that the same thing will happen to me. So, I'm sure that's how it will come up and how we'll explain it.

If the child has any special fears, you would want to allay them as best you can. You can tell them where you will be in the hospital and even show them where the hospital is if they wish to see it and if it is nearby. You may not want to promise that they can visit you when you are in the hospital, unless you are certain this is possible given the hospital's visitor policy and that you will want them there if you do not feel well.

The younger boy went with me to Boston one day, because I was still following up with Dr. X. after the surgery. He sat in on the appointment with me with Dr. X ... But it was kind of strange because he wanted to go up into the hospital to the floor to the room where I was. To this day I don't know why he chose that, but we went to the hospital, because the breast center's right down on the ground. So we went into the hospital. We got in the elevator. We walked around the floor. I showed him where my room was. He was satisfied with that. [Kristen]

Conversely, the surgical experiences of others in the family can be reassuring to children if they turned out well.

They were quite young. I don't think they really understood what potentially could happen. They had seen my mother go through—well, my oldest son was only one, actually, when my mother had surgery. They had seen her post surgery. They didn't really know what she went through. They had heard stories. But they thought, "Well, if Grammy's okay, then Ma's going to be okay." I think they have a sense that that's what you needed to do to stay alive because it worked for Granny. [Valerie]

If the children are very young, say three years old or younger, you may not want to go into detail about your surgery, as they may not understand and may want to concentrate on the issues of absence, i.e., where you will be, for how long (even if they do not have clear sense of time), and caretaking (who will take care of them when you are gone, who will take care of you). Irene spoke about how her young son remembers little of the brief explanation of her PM surgery she gave him at the time.

> Well, my oldest son is just at the age where he's kind of recognizing that women are different than men, so he's very interested in my breasts, which he calls breaffs [phonetic]. He thinks that they're like balloons that it would be fun to pop or something like that, which he doesn't know how close to the truth that really is with implants . . . But, he's not quite at that age where I think he kind of understands what I went through. I mean he knew that I had some surgery and wasn't feeling well and couldn't lift him for a while, but I think that's already erased from his memory and he's moved on. But, certainly, at some point, it will be something that we'll talk to them about and make sure that they understand. [Irene]

Occasionally, a well-meaning parent decides to tell a child a variant of the truth, something which they can understand at their young age, but which is not really true. This is problematic and not advised, since it solves the immediate problem of offering an explanation for an absent and then, an unwell mother, but it can create longer term mistrust if the child remembers that they were told something different from what they later learn is true. Children have powerful antennae for information relating to their parents and they have many opportunities to overhear talk between the parents or between others about the mother's surgery. Thus, it is almost always better to offer truthful advice, even if quite limited, rather than false information.

> Yes, they were too young. I told them that I had to—they were four, and five, five and three, I think they were. They were very into *Madeline* [a popular children's book]. Madeline goes in the hospital and she has her appendix out. So I said that's what I had to have is my appendix out. I would never, you know. I hope that by the time they're my age that I have to start having these conversations, there is just some other cure for it [breast cancer] and it doesn't have to come up. I probably won't ever tell them . . . I just don't want them to have the fear, the fear that it could

happen to them. I'm hoping that by the time it becomes necessary for me to have that conversation that they start to become an age where they should have mammograms and tests, that there's a cure by then. I hope they don't have to know any of this. [Kate]

Sometimes, a parent just thinks that the surgery is not something children should know about at all.

[Tell your children?] No, I don't think I will. I mean with my son, for sure not. With my daughter, someday, well, we'll have to see what's—I don't know. I just don't feel like it's something they even have to be thinking about it. Their mother is already having—I don't think they have to be thinking about their mother's breasts. I don't think it's, you know, for a boy, I don't think it's anything that they have to. If some day this whole issue of the *BRCA1* comes about for them, then we might have to discuss certain things. But just to talk about the fact that I had a prophylactic mastectomy, I don't think that it's any of their business, and I don't think it's within what they should be thinking about. [Harriet]

Obviously, telling older children would involve more details about the surgery and why you chose to have the surgery and why now. Older children might focus quickly on what they will be expected to do in the house to help out with younger children or how your absence might interfere with their plans for social events, etc. It might be important to think about events in their lives, like SAT tests or a prom, etc. in planning the surgery. Daughters might perhaps find news of the surgery more threatening;something which might not be evident at once.

Recently with my daughter, I did. I mean, she's eighteen, and I took her to the gynecologist for the first time. I remember saying to her, "Listen, we don't talk about my operation much, but I want you to know if you have any questions or want to say anything, I want you to feel free to talk about it. It's fine with me" . . . She said to me, well, she just assumed she'll get it, breast cancer. I couldn't believe it. I mean, I didn't know that she even, you know, was thinking like that at all. [Alice]

With children of all ages, you may want to help them understand who they can tell and not tell about your surgery. This can be difficult territory, in that you want your children to have the support of their best friends and some of their parents may already know about your surgery because they are your friends, so they, the friends, may have been told by their parents. However, you may not want it to be a topic of conversation for the entire school or community. This is a reasonable wish to express to children. You may need to help your children know what to say if they are asked by others, both children and adults, outside the circle you wish to share the information with.

My son, I'll definitely, I mean, my sons, I'll definitely tell. It just hasn't really, you know, it's just one of those things. You've got to walk the fine line because I don't mind telling them, but I don't want them to say anything to their friends. [Fay]

ANXIETY

Anxiety in the face of impending surgery is normal, probably close to universal. In retrospect, women told us of many fears related to the surgery which peaked after they had scheduled it, often as the day of the surgery approached, sometimes on the day of surgery. Some were typical fears of individuals who had never had undergone surgery or had been hospitalized. Some women worried about the possible pain.

Well, I was a little nervous, just because it was surgery. But I had total faith in the doctor, and, I don't know, I guess I didn't think much about it. I did, but I didn't, you know? I did know how much pain would be involved, and as it turns out, it wasn't that bad. [Kristen]
It was more private moments of just, I could be driving along in my car and suddenly burst into tears because, again, I was a little scared of what it might be like afterwards. [Fay]

Another woman spoke of being afraid of the anesthesia. She had been told her operation would take six hours and that seemed like a long time to her. She voiced her fears to her surgeon and he reassured her by comparing the experience to taking off and landing an airplane. The risky times with anesthesia were when you were going under and coming out of it and that it did not matter that much how long you were under the anesthesia. Another woman was focused on her fear of needles.

Other women had fears more related to the nature of this surgery. Some spoke about worrying about whether they were doing the right thing. Laura was "very scared going in [to surgery]. I think I was scared, because I thought there was a strong possibility that they would find something." Joyce said, "Of course I was absolutely terrified. Yes, I had really a high level of anxiety. I think more than anything, I was afraid that I was going to be disappointed with the cosmetic result, more than anything else, because I had decided that I wanted them off. The only thing that really calmed me down was that Dr. X said that if I didn't like the result, he could take the implants out." Fay, also, spoke of her worries as surgery approached.

I was scared. Not that I didn't make the right decision. I never let myself think that . . . . I was really worried about was, even though I had totally made this decision on my own and I had lots of time to change my mind if I had wanted to, I was afraid that I wouldn't be as strong or wonderful about how I felt about myself afterwards. I mean, I had a plan that I was going to feel great about it and that I knew I did the right thing and I was going to love my new body no matter what it looked like. But I thought, well, what if I'm saying all that and then I wake up and I have a completely different reaction? That worried me. Those are my, I think, yes, my two biggest fears. Fortunately, I woke up and, fortunately, I was able to handle the whole thing as well or better than I had hoped.

Prophylactic mastectomy is elective, yet major, surgery. A woman will never know if she would have developed breast cancer without the surgery. Several women in our study spoke of this thought as they approached the day of surgery. We asked women if they had had a moment where they felt like changing their minds before surgery and a few talked about last minute hesitation: "Oh, yes," Harriet told us. "I mean I kind of did, yes. You never know if you're making the right decision. It's a very hard decision. So, no one comes and tells you that this is the right thing. You never know if it's necessary or not."

THE DAY OF SURGERY

When the day of her prophylactic mastectomy finally came for Irene, she felt a mixture of fear and elation.

I had a really hard time walking into the hospital. That was probably the hardest moment. Once I made up the decision and spent the five months thinking about it and whatever, but actually going into the hospital, and you go into the prep room. Right before they gave me any kind of sedative, I did panic a little bit, and I said, "Boy, you know you don't really have to do this." I started to have second doubts.

We walked to the hospital. "How do you feel?" "Oh, my God. What have I done? What am I doing?" But, you know, that's what you want to do, so you do it. I think going in I was certainly nervous about it, but also kind of excited and relieved that I was finally getting to the day where I was going to have this done and get it behind me. So, that was good. [Kate]

THE RIGHT CHOICE, BUT NOT AN IDEAL OPTION

And, finally, there is the reality that prophylactic mastectomy is not the ultimate, ideal solution for prevention of breast cancer in high risk women; it is only an interim solution, until something less invasive can be found. This balanced view of one patient reflected her feeling that is was a choice, but not a truly ideal choice.

I didn't feel like I had a choice in this at all. I felt like this was something I had to do, I had to deal with, I would have felt worse had I gotten cancer and not have done something more severe to stop it. So I didn't really feel like I made a decision. It was more like it was just something I really had to do. I couldn't live my life like that anymore with that feeling of impending doom. I don't want to. Personally, I would like to see the medical community find a cure. To do surgery like this seems kind of barbaric, but given all the options at the time, this one seemed like the smartest choice. [Kate]

CHAPTER 5

Surgery

Surgery is never an easy process, but it is often hard to anticipate just how it will be difficult. For women who have decided to undergo a prophylactic mastectomy (PM), it seems that the decision is often experienced in a rather cerebral way (albeit involving many emotional factors). The decision is so much a matter of weighing many options without the roaring, urgent tiger of breast cancer behind one to raise adrenaline levels and encourage certainty that it almost seems shocking when the surgery actually happens. There are so many details to learn and contrast. A woman becomes an expert on the reconstructive options available and, in so doing, becomes numb to the reality that a surgeon will cut into her body, causing her pain, and leaving a body both in need of healing and at risk for infection. When words are transformed into action, the shock of this transition can be heard in the voices of some of the women in our study as they spoke about their postsurgical awakening.

The recovery from surgery is both a physical and an emotional process. The emotional is a much stronger component of the recovery from PM than the recovery following surgery on an internal organ, such as liver, kidney, or gall bladder. In PM surgery, the changes are, at least for most women, heavily laden with meaning related to femininity and sense of self, and have great interpersonal ramifications. But the physical component—the "pains and drains"—cannot be quickly dismissed. In this chapter, we will consider the physical and emotional components of recovery from PM surgery for women who have never been diagnosed with cancer. We will talk about the process of returning to normal or the "new normal" and of how that goal was reached by different women.

IMMEDIATELY AFTER SURGERY—"PAINS AND DRAINS"

The moment of awakening from PM surgery is an enormous physical and emotional milestone. A woman has accomplished that which has been planned, often for years. But the immediate physical reality is not likely to be a pleasant one in which to contemplate the meaning of the moment. The pain, as in any surgery, is real and must be continually assessed and contained. Immediate physical limitations are also real. A woman has gone from being healthy and without restriction to a state of temporary unwellness. For many women, these are difficult moments.

Janice says, "I didn't think I'd be as sick as I was. You do get sick afterwards. That's the only thing, I think. I had no pain." Laura remembers that her early recovery was:

[h]orrible. I had no clue how bad I would feel. I had reactions to the pain [medicine] and couldn't stop vomiting. For the entire days I was there, it was terrible. The pain was horrible. It was much, much worse than I would have ever guessed. . . . But the really horrible pain, I'm trying to remember. It seems like it was a long time. I know I went back for my checkup when they took the drains out. At that point I couldn't even walk. I could walk, I could say, but I couldn't walk the distance from in the hall of the hospital. I was put in a wheelchair. I mean I was really feeling terrible . . . But the recovery was pretty intense. Those first four days in the hospital were pretty painful, and I can remember being in so much pain that I couldn't watch TV because I couldn't simulate [sic] looking at them and hearing the words and putting it together. It took like three days to be able to do that. So, yes, it was interesting.

With preparation about what postsurgery would feel like, Meredith was able to anticipate some of her reaction and she formulated an image that helped carry her through those first days.

No, I kind of knew it was going to be like that. No, I mean . . . , because I had had that woman to talk to and she had told me it's a lot more rugged than they let on that it is. So, yes, I was expecting. I actually went home from the hospital a day sooner than I was supposed to . . . I looked at it [recovery] as if, when I was a kid, I grew up on a lake, and I'm a swimmer. I just looked at it like that. It was the weirdest thing. One morning you would get up early and you're perfectly healthy and you drive down to Boston and you walk into this hospital, you're feeling fine. It's like you're diving into a lake and you've got a long, long ways to go before you hit the surface again, and then you've still got to swim all the way to the other side . . . And I just kept visualizing that and six weeks down the road I was still sort of human again . . . Still it is, it's a three month, if you do TRAM flap, it's a good three months of recovery, and it's really a year before you really feel good again. You're tired for a year. But I still think that it's going to be better than wondering if you—I mean I couldn't imagine what it would be like having that kind of recovery and also going through chemotherapy and waiting to find out how you were staged and seeing if it spread and wondering if it's coming back and all that. I still feel as though I had it easier.

Chantal had an easier time than many women after the PM surgery, which she attributed to her doctor's skill.

I was a little nervous, but nothing overwhelming. You know, I did my normal nesting, making sure everything was ready for everybody. I thought it was going to be a lot worse than it was. . . . I still think I really lucked out with the surgeon I had. She had the opportunity to use this wonderful stuff where they put it inside you. I guess, they use it on heart patients or something. And it numbs you. I mean, I'm just finally after two years getting the feeling back, but it was great. I had no pain. It numbs you from the inside so you heal better and—because I have talked to other people that had the surgery, and they said it was very painful, and mine wasn't. . . . I had the surgery and I was weak the next day. I went home. I was teaching at the time. I stayed out of school for a week and was back teaching.

Hanna found the postsurgery period to be a moment in which many things came together for her. It was a meaningful milestone for her and for her husband.

When I woke up from surgery, I hurt like hell. Then, you probably think I'm crazy, but I remember my husband was so sweet. When I woke up, he gave me a new diamond, an anniversary diamond, and it was gorgeous. To me, it was the sweetest thing. He told me, he said, "This is for new beginnings, Hanna, since you're not going to have to worry no more." I thought that was nice.

But the weird thing is that when I was knocked out and when I was like starting to come to, I felt my mother's presence with me. I felt like my mother said, "Hanna, you did the right thing. Don't worry about it. You're going to be fine." That kind of spooked me, because I'd never felt my mother's presence prior to that for a long time. But I felt like she was there and she told me I'm going to be okay. So that was weird, and, basically, I haven't shared that with too many people because I don't want people thinking I'm nuts. I know that she was there and I know that she, whatever. . . . I felt that after she had done that, I knew everything was going to be okay.

TAKING THE BANDAGES OFF THE FIRST TIME

While awakening from the anesthesia, a woman physically feels the pain of surgery. The first time the surgical bandages are removed and the wound is dressed, the visual effects are apparent to her. Women spoke of this as a turning point in their relationship to their breasts and bodies. Strong words, like "freak" or "Frankenstein" were used not infrequently about their initial reactions, although, as with Rose below, retrospectively, the changes since surgery often countered those difficult first images.

I looked like the woman from *Night of the Living Dead*. If you really think about it, what they do is they rearrange your upper chest, so you really do look horrid, but it's amazing over time how remarkably better it looks. As far as the bandages it looks very shocking. It's good that people see pictures beforehand. Breast tissue is not just your breast, it's also your clavicle. Also it's a different quality of breast, it's something about it being too thin. The scar also looks really bad, but then over time it really vanishes, especially if you have a really good plastic surgeon.

I have to tell you, what I first saw, it was better than I thought it was going to be [when bandages were first removed]. The same thing with my husband. We were both, because I was able to, if I just lifted my hands up and just covered the incisions, it really looked like normal breasts. There was a comforting thought in that. Incisions are terrible, but they do, scars fade. I knew that that would be better over time, and, in fact, they have been. But, when I saw it for the first time, it wasn't awful. I thought it would be worse than it was ... There was a lot of adjusting, definitely. I also have to say that I'm somebody who beforehand I had really quite a heavy breast. I was more like a D, which I really hated. So, when I did the surgery, I asked for B cups, and there was a little bit of improvement on the whole. [Sandra]

I remember, even though I knew essentially what it would look like, because my sister had been through that and I had helped her, it's still kind of shocking to have the bandages come off and have nothing there anymore. So, yes, kind of a little shocking, but still I was very convinced that I was doing the right thing, so I was able to deal with it. ... I don't think I shed any tears over the loss of the breast tissue. I wanted it gone ... But, I think I was pleased that I had the reconstruction done, and I think that helped kind of ease the transition because I was still going in periodically to have my expanders filled and get to the right size and then having the surgery where my implants were actually put in. I think just kind of following through with all of that kind of helped. It was kind of a sense of rebuilding what had been lost, and that helped. So, I feel very much myself now with the implants, and it's been an okay transition. [Irene]

The narratives also illustrate the significant impact supportive people can have at such vulnerable moments in a woman's life.

It was a little bit shocking because everything was still bruised, a little swollen. But I kind of looked at it with the viewpoint of knowing my husband took me the way I was, my kids gave me the support, that people were there. If I had had a problem or questions or whatever, I could always pick up a phone to talk with somebody. That really kind of made me feel a little—it was a little shocking for me the first time because I had to accept it. But I accepted it in a positive, not a negative. I think with my husband saying he didn't care, he didn't care how I looked, as long as I was okay with myself. [Janice]

In one case, however, the narratives illustrated the high emotional cost which someone can exact who is not sensitive to the critical transition of this moment. Julia recounted a difficult time she had with the resident who did the dressing change the first time.

> As soon as Dr. X's nurse practitioner came up, I said, "You know, I am strong as an ox," and I said, "I'm very comfortable with my decision, but if somebody really wanted to test me, it was the resident who took down my dressing." I said, "I did go and look after he left, and it looks pretty scary." I said, "I can't believe I see my ribs so much. I look like one of those poor African children with the potbellies and then their ribs showing"... My ribs were— I mean you can count my ribs, because I'm kind of pear-shaped. But, I said, "Somebody has to have a long talk with him," I said, "because it was the most horrible experience and it made me feel like such a freak, without a doubt." I said, "Well, there it is. A man saying, 'Boy, honey, you look a mess.'" So, I was devastated.

WHAT IS DIFFICULT AND WHAT HELPS

The physical recovery after a PM, like any postsurgical recovery, is a slow process, aided if possible by recommended exercise, often accompanied by pain, and requiring a significant dose of patience. Women were eager to offer suggestions for what had been helpful to them through this period. Kristen felt researching the likely aftereffects was her way of gaining mastery over the anticipated postsurgical unpleasantries.

> Oh, yes. I'm not the kind of person who deals with ignorance as bliss. I'm better off, the more I know. The more I know, the better off I am ... Yes, in fact, I would say that anybody who's considering this [having a PM], if they don't do research and aren't that interested in finding out all they can, I would be a little leery of them. You know what I mean?

But finding information for women who had a prophylactic mastectomy (as opposed to mastectomy following a cancer diagnosis) was not so easy, as Meredith observed.

> Yes [a book helped], but they weren't for people like me who had done the prophylactic. They were people that had the mastectomy

and had had reconstruction . . . They were anecdotes from people
who had done it and how they all seemed to experience this thing
where they would show off their boobs like a new car, you know.
So you became sort of like an exhibitionist for about a year. But
maybe, like I said, it was different if I wasn't someone who was
going to have it prophylactically done. If it was someone who
had just gotten breast cancer, maybe then it would be helpful,
because you'd think then you'd have to know how to tell people
and be prepared for their reactions.

Fay offered suggestions about pain management, exercise, and
about the importance of humor in recovery.

So what would happen, I had a little booklet that was given to me
at the hospital that talked about things like range of motion, and
things I could be doing when I got home to help my recovery. . . .
So I discovered a little trick and I always pass this along to the
other women that I speak with when I get referral calls. But what
I would do is—as I say, this was like my little routine—I'd wake
up in the morning, take a Tylenol with codeine. I'd take just
one; and then I'd go in the shower and I'd let all that hot water
kind of loosen me up a little bit. But also because the pain pill also
took a little edge off because it always seemed to hurt more when
I first woke up in the morning. . . . And it hurt a lot initially, so
that by taking that pill, it enabled me to kind of work a little bit
beyond the pain. What I would do in the shower, I would just
walk my fingers up the walls of the showers. I would kind of have
my own benchmarks with that so that each day I could see my
own improvement of being able to reach a little or stretch a little
higher. So by that time, a month had gone by.
   We talk very openly about it [the PM surgery], and it is
something—this is one of the major things I really want to get
across today is that humor—humor is the *numero uno* tool for
healing, to get an understanding amongst people that you live
with, that you work with, that you hang around with, people in
your community. Having and approaching the whole thing with
a sense of openness and humor is a great educational tool, and
it's also quite selfishly a way of getting them to treat you the same
as they did before—and not look at you like you're some kind of
oddity, or feel sorry for you or anything like that. That, the way
I started doing it, immediately after I got home from my surgeries,

was I would make jokes about it with people so that they would feel comfortable with me. . . . Humor was definitely a way to get through the whole thing.

Meredith said that daily exercise helped, but also spoke about how difficult the physical recovery was for her.

But I knew the best thing to do would be to walk, so I just started walking probably two weeks after the surgery I started going on walks. It was hard because I didn't have a lot of blood so I was breathing hard. I hired a cleaning service to come in and clean my house. I had my kids back by then, and I hired a babysitter to come in every day and watch my kids for about three hours, and I would walk about two miles down to a lake. Then I'd do stretching exercises in the lake, which seemed easier, and then I'd walk two miles back again. It would hurt and sting and I'd be crouched, but it seemed like the walking seemed to help me stretch out. But it was hard. It was a hard recovery process.

Joyce relied on expertise that she had available about diet and yoga to help her recovery.

When I was recovering from my surgery, I had private yoga classes in which my yoga instructor and I went over all of the sore places on my body, and we worked on those sore places to get my flexibility back. My flexibility came back in ten days, and I think that's a record. On the nutrition end, because I had three Ph.D.s in nutrition and four dieticians who I have here at my disposal at _____ University here telling me what to eat around my surgery. I think I'm not wrong in saying I broke the record for getting drains out after the mastectomy. Their record was four days, and mine were ready to come out in two days. On average, women have their drains in for seven days. I'm convinced that it's because I was eating a diet that was designed for me by wound care specialists and nutritionists.

Other women in our study found that swimming or massage were helpful to their recovery.

I'll tell you one thing that really did a tremendous help for me postoperatively after a few months was massage therapy. After the initial time of telling the person, "I have a lot of scars, they do not hurt," but going into it with them knowing what my condition was before they did it. They did a fantastic [job] both mental and physical, because they relaxed muscles in my back, and mentally because they didn't scream in horror and just me go off into gaga land, you know [Ingrid].

Familial support and wanting to look healthy for one's children were also mentioned as important factors in speeding recovery. Irene recalled, "Yes, but they were both very good [my kids], and, like I said, I had a lot of family support around the house in the weeks after the surgery. So, that made it must easier." Hanna told of the hard times and the value of support: "I can't lie. I would be lying to you if I said, "Yes, there was no. I went through it with smiles all the way." No, that's not true. I think everybody that goes through it, like with any surgery, you go for a while and then you hit bottom. Then you climb right back up. I think if you have the right support, then you can get through it." Julie talked proudly of needing less time in the hospital.

I was shocked at how easy the recovery period was, because I had watched my mother with mastectomies, and I had watched tons of women because I used to do general surgery. I really feel that it is an attitude. I just got up the next day and said, "I'm going to brush my hair whether it hurts or not." A, I didn't want everybody to know I had two mastectomies, so I thought, well, I have to really be moving here pretty good. My immediate family did, I mean all my kids did and everything, and I spoke about it. But, no, I was ready to go home in twenty-four hours. I wanted to get out of the hospital. She [my doctor] offered me a second night because my insurance covered it. I think most people should have a second night because I do think it is a lot. But I wanted to get home for my children and show them I was fine.

Psychological counseling after PM was the key to recovery for some women.

I did end up into counseling afterwards. I did seek out a therapist to talk to regarding it [the PM]. Basically, I came to terms with it when she said to me, "Well, basically, Debbie, who has a perfect body?" When I looked, and I sat and I thought, I said, "Well, yes, that's true." Because she said, "As a woman, we always want to have something we don't have. Some of us want a flat stomach, some of us want bigger thighs, some of us want smaller breasts or bigger breasts." She said, "None of us are ever really happy with what we have. So what is the perfect body? Describe it." I couldn't do it, so therefore, I came to terms with it. Really, none of us do have perfect bodies, and we always want what we can't have. [Hanna]

EMOTIONAL ADJUSTMENTS

Me–Not Me

The reintegration of a woman's self-concept and body image following PM surgery is an important aspect of her emotional recovery. These changes are reflected in women's statements about their feelings regarding the loss of their natural breasts and their revised bodies. The evolution over time of this reintegration means that women are at different places at different times on the Me-Not Me dichotomy in relation to their breasts. A woman's concept of her femininity and the role her breasts play in that conceptualization led women who had undergone PM to quite different conclusions about the impact of surgery. Some women felt the loss of their breasts quite acutely, while others expressed positive reactions towards what they saw as an improvement in their appearance.

Women's thoughts about modesty in relation to showing their breasts to others also reflect their integration of the "new normal." Modesty reflects not only a woman's basic beliefs about showing her body, but in her postsurgical life, it reflects her feelings about her new body, without her natural breasts, and either without reconstruction or with her newly constructed breasts or breasts-in-progress. This sense of modesty affects intimate contacts with her husband or lover, decisions about undressing in front of her children, ways of acting in dressing or locker rooms, and sometimes, decisions about showing her breasts to people more distant in relationship.

While this adjustment process occurs for all women who have a mastectomy, women undergoing PM know that the surgery was not an absolute medical necessity. Ultimately, it was a personal choice about the management of risk. As such, women's feelings about the surgical outcomes have an even larger imprint on their self-evaluation. These women chose this surgery. A good or at least acceptable outcome reinforces the woman's sense that she can take good care of herself, that she can process difficult, complex information and make good choices.

THE LOSSES: WAKING UP IS HARD TO DO

Hanna's words conveyed the challenges she experienced in facing herself and seeing her changed body immediately after surgery. She ably described the process of trying to come to acceptance and the conscious messages she gave herself in that effort.

[When bandages were removed] I said, "Oh, what did I do?" It was hard. I don't know. They looked like breasts, for being without. I think it was probably the roundness thing. They looked like breasts, they moved like breasts, they bounced and they were symmetric and everything was even and they looked fine. They were smaller, which was nice. I missed the part that the nipples are not like what nipples are. I don't like the fact that the areola, it's not a true color, as you would say that they were. The nipple area is very, very—it's not. They don't look real. Other than that, my breasts look as real as can be. You can hardly tell where the scars were, and they look great. But it's just the nipple area, you can tell they're not real. That bothers me, but nobody sees me but my husband.

Yes, I miss the sensation, and I wish I had better nipples, because I'm not pleased with it. But as far as feeling like I'm attractive and a woman, yes, I am, because I walk down the street and I still have guys looking at me. So I feel good. I'm very happy, because I'm still a woman.

For Hanna, this transformation was not without its emotional costs. She admits to being quite depressed as she adjusted to her new body.

I'd wake up, cry every day. I didn't feel complete, didn't feel whole. I felt people knew but didn't know. I was almost paranoid. I felt like I couldn't do anything, because at that time I really had no feeling to the breast at all. Because of the type of work that I'm in, taking care of babies, and when they pinch you, you, basically, feel it. But sometimes I'd get pinched in the breast and I wouldn't feel it until they'd black and blue me. That would bother me, that I did not feel complete for a while. I felt like I was deformed in some way . . . Basically, I know to a woman their breasts are very sexual and it's a part of their sexuality, and, yes, it is. But, again, it's not who makes us, it's not what makes us. I know that it is the part of us that makes us different from men, but, again, it's not who I am. It's not what makes me . . . who I am. It's a part of me.

Other women spoke of the losses they felt after the PM surgery.

I think they felt I was—you know, I miss my breasts dearly, and I do feel like less of a woman. There's a whole part, but I'd rather be less of a woman and be here than dealing with all the garbage I saw my mother and other women deal with. I think until you're in that circumstance, it's like you don't know about how it is to have a child until you have a child. You know, you have to be there. No one can really support you in the way you need. [Julia]

I'll tell you the truth, the person it most affects . . . in my experience, the person it most affects is yourself. You would think your spouse and this and that. But the truth is everyone else can kind of live with it, and the hardest one is on yourself . . . Yes, it's with you all the time. I mean I can't say for everyone, but what I found is your spouse loves you and then they adjust and you can make it so you're attractive to them, but it's yourself that you have to learn to look at it's very important how you view yourself. You have to learn to look at yourself as normal and healthy, so that's like a struggle. [Harriet]

For some women, the transformation recaptured feelings of being a young girl or created feelings of having a body which more closely resembled that of a boy or man.

"You look just like a mannequin, a store mannequin, and it didn't have the correct shape. It had nothing on it." [Ingrid]

"Oh, yes. I still look at myself in the mirror, and I kind of chuckle, because I look like I did at eleven." [Julia]

"It was like having breasts of a 37-year-old woman going down to a 16-year-old woman again. I was like, whoa." [Hanna]

"THEY'RE GORGEOUS": POSITIVE OUTCOMES

Women do sometimes feel elated about the breasts that have been reconstructed for them and feel that their looks have improved post-surgery. The self-confidence which results may be due to both the absence of worry about a body which previously was, as some say, not to be trusted, and the freedom to enjoy their breasts and the effects the women perceive them as having on others.

Oh, yes, the very first thing I did, of course, was check and make sure [unclear] look down. What do I look like? He had put implants in, the stretchers in. Now, I was never very big breasted anyways, so that the stretchers were about the size of my original size any how. So I really didn't notice a difference. Body image wise and everything, I was absolutely fine. My girlfriend walked in and she looked at me, and she said, "I don't see any difference." She laughed and she said, "In fact, they may even be a little bigger." [Sandra]

I don't know that I really thought anything of it, other than I didn't feel like I was less a person. The avenue that some people go down, I didn't feel that at all. I don't hold a strong thing for that. It wasn't like I was missing anything. Some people do, but I'm not. I don't go there. [Vicky]

That's very much an upside of it. To be honest with you, I think they're nicer than the originals, so I get more admiring glances now than I ever did before the surgery. I wear tight sweaters, and I show them off, because they look good. What percentage of the world knows they're not real, so I flaunt them, really. I'll be real honest about it, I flaunt them because they're gorgeous. . . . I think it's easier for me to say that I compare the relationship I had with my old breasts with the relationship I have with my new breasts.

The relationship I had with my old breasts was an acrimonious relationship. We weren't really fond of each other in the sense that I always had a feeling that they were going to really kill me some day. So I was never particularly attached to them, because from a very young age I had learned to be very suspicious of them. I did monthly breast self-examinations in which they were on one side and I was on the other side. Do you sort of understand what it is I'm trying to say? These breasts I have a much better relationship with because not only do they look good and have a nice shape, I know they're not going to turn on me. They're much more welcome on my chest than were my original breasts because they look good and, as I say—let me see. A friend of mine who's a lawyer and a real wit said, "The other ones were booby traps." [Joyce]

One of the interesting aspects of the outcomes of prophylactic mastectomy is that there are often both negative and positive

outcomes expressed by the same woman. This seems realistic given
the intense preparation, the sense of loss and the simultaneous perception of seizing control of a fearful circumstance, and eliminating
or vastly reducing the threat through self-imposed surgery. It is critical
that we hear both sides from women. Some research studies show an
absence of regret about the PM decision,[1, 2] but this does not mean that
there may not be real feelings of loss and sadness at having to undergo
surgery and having to think about cancer risk at a young age due to
hereditary predisposition. There are also deep satisfactions which we
will consider in greater depth in subsequent chapters.

MIXED OUTCOMES: LOSSES AND POSITIVES

Introduction: A True Picture of the Impact of PM Includes the Gains and Losses

I don't mean to minimize, but there is still loss. You're losing
your breast, you're losing an extremely important part of who
you are, and your sexuality. So, I don't mean to minimize that.
But there were some pluses in that, I mean, I even still feel that
today. I'm always happy. My family, we just took a long walk
and we were on scooters, and I thought, I still think, "Oh, I don't
need to wear a bra." I don't have to strap myself in one of those
armor-plated bras to do any sports. . . . I think all of us have different relationships with our breasts.
    I think it might be difficult for somebody who really felt very,
very positively about her breasts, that they were very beautiful
parts of her body. I didn't really. I always felt that they were just
too big for my body. There was a slight embarrassment about
having D cup, so, oddly enough, that sort of played in my favor
in making it less of a loss than it might have been . . . Yes, I mean
there was definitely sort of a loss, even though, as I said, I wasn't
crazy about my breasts, they were my breasts. They had, you
know, they were part of who I was as a sexual being, and that
was a real adjustment to have to. I mean that was a real loss.
There is no doubt about that. [Sandra]

MODESTY/IMMODESTY

With modern reconstructive surgery or breast prostheses, women do
not have to fear that, when dressed in their normal clothes, anyone

would be able to guess that they had had their breasts removed. However, in the intimate setting of one's bedroom, in normal day-to-day circumstances within one's immediate family, or, for some women, in settings like dressing or locker rooms, the effects of prophylactic mastectomy may be more obvious. Women spoke with feeling about this level of integration of their new bodies.

With Husbands and Lovers

Julia spoke quite specifically about how affected she was by her memories of her mother's mastectomy and its aftermath, and her feelings of being less attractive following her surgery and how they both played in to her interactions with her husband.

It wasn't until we went away this past May. I said, "I haven't really walked across the room nude in front of you."

He goes, "I've noticed."

Not that I did it all the time, but if we were on vacation, it was just—it was—I said, "I don't want to repulse you."

He said, "You don't repulse me." He goes, "You look different. I am not going to tell you that you don't look different." But he said, "It's you." And he goes, "So, you're my little girl now." He's very cute about it, but I still—and he's never winced at all. He will always hug me, and right after my surgery he would say, "When can I wrap my arms around you? I don't want to hurt you."

I'd make cracks like, "Well, there's nothing there. Why do you want to?"

He'd punch me and go, "Because it's you and I like to hug you." So, I think that that must be very important. I mean I know it's very important, and I can't imagine if women don't have that kind of support because it's taken me two years to kind of feel comfortable in my own skin, and he's been there from the beginning.

I remember my mother saying about my father, "Oh, he can't even hold me or look at me." That scarred me. She probably should have never said that to me, but I remember that . . . You could see the agony in her eyes.

I guess I feel worse for my husband than I feel for myself because I'm not the person I was, you know, physically. There's just no way you can escape. It's like being an amputee. It's a horrible, and I had with all the support in the world, I still feel like I'm half a woman, but I'm still comfortable in my own skin.

With Children

Children living at home are, of course, aware of their mother's surgery and are typically also curious about the changes in her body. They are also often quite frank in their appraisals.

> I obviously don't parade around fully naked. I obviously don't do that. I also don't feel that I have to go and get changed behind closed doors or anything, especially with my kids. That was probably one of the things I worried about. I thought if I don't feel comfortable undressing in front of my children, what does that say about how I feel about my body? I would say I was a little concerned about that. But I have found that I can undress in front of them, and I don't feel like I have to cover everything up. I feel like if I'm just modest enough that I can do that. [Kate]
>
> Well, when I first had it done and she was really little, I think I was insecure myself. I felt like I should show it to her because I wanted the kids' natural reaction, that, here. [Laughing] You know, after I finished the entire reconstruction and everything, I'd show her. I remember, like, I think she was little surprised I'd done something like this, like, "What did you do?" You know, I didn't get much reaction. She didn't, and I said, "Well, so what do you think they look like?" Then I remember her saying at the time, "Pepperonis." [Laughter] Since then I haven't, I don't undress in front of her. We're kind of a modest family, you know. [Alice]

Dressing Rooms and Locker Rooms

We asked women if they had any special feelings now when in a locker or dressing room, places where women typically undress in front of other women. Julia told us, "Yes, when you go into those big dressing rooms, I'm very quick to get dressed, and, of course, I'd never take off my bra. Yes, I do. I'm wondering if people can tell. And I do, I feel like a freak. There is part of me that feels like a freak." Janice similarly said, "I usually do, yes. I usually do [feel uncomfortable getting undressed]. What I do is just like when I shower, I just get dressed behind the door or something like that. I always make sure I was dressed in some way. I would never just come out of a dressing room with a towel or something like that." Rose concurred in a different way, "No, I feel like I could shrug off my clothes in the locker room and that's fine. What I do find, and it makes me self-conscious, is only times when I get a massage. I'm usually a private person, so I find instances like that kind of awkward."

Life in this respect was also altered for Beth and Sandra. "I never go in a public dressing room. I'm pretty careful about it," Beth said. "If I'm at the gym, I take a shower in the, you know, I don't take it in the public. I go in the private, and I never get massages or anything like that, but I never did before either." Sandra, when asked how she felt about locker room encounters said:

> I mean I'm in a college, and we've got the campus locker rooms. And I would never take my shirt off, I mean, be bare breasted. I mean there are other students and other faculty, and I think that's just way too much to lay on the unsuspecting public in a sense. So, if I use the locker room, I go into the bathroom when I need to change my top, and that's sad. I'm sorry about that. Last summer we spent six weeks in France, and everybody's walking around without a top. I can't, even if I'd wanted to, which I don't know ... I've never done it before, but I certainly wouldn't ever even conceive of doing it now.

On the other end of the spectrum, Chantal, however, said "I'm as comfortable as I would normally be changing in a dressing room in front of strangers."

A Single Woman's Experience

Our sample of women who had undergone bilateral PM included only one single woman. This is likely not accidental or a sampling error. More married women seek PM for a multiplicity of reasons— some financial, some emotional, and interpersonal. Married women are more likely to feel they have a supportive, understanding spouse whom they can count on for support before, during, and after surgery. They are likely to have their childbearing years behind them and, therefore, are not concerned about losing the opportunity to breast-feed children. And, likely, many single women, like Joyce, worry how their dating and sexual relationships would be affected by PM.

> I think that's a really interesting question because I've been trying to figure it out myself [how PM affects sexual attractiveness/ desire]. First, I'm single. I wanted to see how it was—at the time

I made the decision, I was going out with a guy, but we didn't have that close of a relationship. In fact, I was thinking of ending the relationship anyway, but I sort of used him as a guinea pig to try out his response to my surgery. I think his very positive response and the fact that he was supportive about it, and that he still really wanted to go out with me after the surgery and that it was my decision to end the relationship was very good for me psychologically.

I have actively not dated for the last year, because my breasts really were kind of shocking looking, I would think, for somebody who is seeing them for the first time. The reconstruction wasn't finished. I probably could have gone through the reconstruction and the nipple reconstruction faster than I did, but I was sort of trying to put it in around my teaching schedule and other demands of work.

I've never actually taken these [her breasts] out sexually in public, and I've never actually shown them to a man that I'm dating. How would I feel about that? I don't think I would have liked to have done that before the nipple reconstruction was done. I've had the nipple reconstructed now, and in January I'm getting the tattooing [of the nipples] done. I think at this point I'm ready to take them out into public in the sense that I wouldn't mind, at this point, showing them to a man that I'm having a sexual relationship with. I think they were so shocking looking when they just had the sutures across them. I think that that's not a big deal for your husband, but if it's somebody you're dating and you don't have a close relationship with, I certainly wouldn't want to shock them with it. So I just decided not to go that route or even to take them out in public before then.

So in that sense, yes, I've held back my sex life. I have had many offers to go to bed by men over this last year that know they're dealing with saline implants. If I've turned them down, it's been for other reasons, not because they weren't willing. I guess I've learned a lot about men and how they respond to this, and I think for single women this is really important. This is very important. The only one possibly negative thing was from a guy that I considered being completely spineless anyway, and I just wanted to see if I was right in thinking that he would completely disappear off my dating map because I'd only been out with him a few times. He called and said, "Hi, where have you been? Haven't heard from you for a long time?" I said, "Oh, I've had some surgery." He said, "Oh, well, what kind of surgery?" I said, "Well, as a matter of fact, I had a prophylactic mastectomy." I thought, "Okay, let's see how he deals with it." I was absolutely right in thinking that. He never called me back again. I think a lot of women would worry. The thing is that I talk to my cousins and I look at their family history and I'm trying to measure. They've had their kids. They've finished with breastfeeding. The only thing that happens to their breasts now is that they get saggier. I guess my feeling is having made this decision as a single woman, I look at my married cousins and I think, "My God, what are you waiting for? Why, if it wasn't so overwhelmingly difficult for a woman like me who's single and actively dates men and has to take these things out in public, you've just got a husband and you've been married for fifteen or twenty years, what is the big deal? Just go get them cut off. Why are you waiting for, a breast cancer diagnosis?" I'm wondering if, for them, the issue isn't the sexual aspects of breasts and whether they wouldn't find sex less enjoyable having their breasts off. But I can't answer that question for them.

Showing Others

A number of women dealt with their new breasts as if they were not intimate body parts, at least initially. They were eager to show them off to colleagues and friends and even sons to illustrate how remarkable the surgery was in creating relatively natural-looking breasts or in illustrating the changes that removal without reconstruction yielded.

No, basically, people laugh because I say I have no modesty, [unclear] they are not me. They are just there, so there's nothing to be modest about anymore. As far as letting anybody that I worked with or something, if they really wanted to see what a reconstruction looked like, why, sure, I don't care. Come up to the lounge, and I'll show you. I have no modesty at all. [Emily]

But, you know, it's funny. In the beginning, I don't know why, but for the first year or two, first of all, all my friends wanted to see them, and you don't even feel like they're yours, so you show them. You start to show everybody your boobs. I can remember one Thanksgiving when all women went in the bathroom to see them. And they all liked them better than theirs because, you know, we've all had kids and these are very perky ... I'm less likely now to show someone my breasts. They feel more like they belong to me and less like I bought them at a store. In the beginning they felt like something I got. I don't know. I mean I can't say that I was ever traumatized by it, you know. It's what I expected, and actually I'm much happier with the results than the pictures that I saw. [Meredith]

When he [my son] came home one day after the surgery was over and done with, he asked me a few questions about it, and I said to him, "Well, do you want to see my chest, because maybe someday you may have to see something like this with a girlfriend or a wife or whatever?" You know, my scars didn't really look that bad, and I thought, you know, I gave him opportunity to see it, if he wanted to. This is the oldest boy. He didn't want to see it, but he wanted to feel it. I remember I had a tee shirt on at the time, no bra. So I stood in front and he ran his hand down my chest and you could feel my ribs. My chest is like a washboard, because you can feel every rib. He just was kind of amazed and he said, "I can feel all your ribs." I said, "Yes." I said, "That's it. They're gone." So he was curious about that. So he felt it, but he didn't want to see it. [Kristen]

RESIDUAL RISK

While prophylactic mastectomy drastically reduces the chances that a high risk woman will have breast cancer, it does not eliminate all such risk. The underlying tissue may, in rare cases, harbor cancer cells which, with time, become tumors. In our interviews, we asked women how they dealt with knowing they still had some residual risk of getting breast cancer.

No, because I felt like Dr. X was being very truthful with me. I mean, nobody could guarantee that that's 100 percent. You know, she could leave cells behind, and who knows? If she'd said to me that, "This is 100 percent guaranteed that you're not going to get breast cancer," I would have looked at her kind of funny, you know, because I'd think to myself, how can she say that? She's not God. But she said, she told me right off that this was not 100 percent. She could never say it was 100 percent, so that, to me, was even more reassuring because she was being so straight with me . . . I have myself checked about every six-eight months. Well, if it happens, it happens. I did everything I could. [Kristen]

Oh, it's, well, they basically told me that there's no way I can get breast cancer. Now, there're certainly other types of cancer that one can worry about and other [unclear] cancer that have been in my family, although not majorly so [unclear] colon cancer. But, I mean, it's just I don't think about it very much, I guess. I just try to eat well and to hope for the best . . . They talked about it as there was none. I had a little trouble with that because I know that there's some skin that I have, and I have, and a little bit of skin, that was part of my old breast that's still there. You know, I wonder about it sometimes to myself now, and occasionally ask that question again of different doctors that I meet along the way . . . You know, I don't have breasts anymore, so I don't have—they'll do mammograms, and I have asked my regular family doctor, "Do you feel, like, under my armpit to feel, does that—."

He goes, "Well, yes, you could get all kinds of—you know, people get cancer in different lymph glands that are in different parts of your body. But the chances of you getting it now are certainly slimmer. [Fay]"

It certainly—you know, I think it was disappointing to think, well, I can't just eliminate this from my life altogether. But at the same time, I recognized that by, you know, with a good surgeon and getting rid of as much breast tissue as I could, that I really was reducing my risk down to just what the general population has, or maybe a little below that even. That, for me, was a substantial step. I mean that was a large reduction of risk, compared with what I was faced with at the time I made the decision to have the surgery. So, like I said, I wished I could have done more, but this just seemed like the right step and a good step. [Irene]

Rose told us that she was informed about the residual risk, but she felt that the odds were a lot less, and that she would actually, if she ever did get anything back, or anything recurred, she would feel like she had done everything she possibly could. She described it like a flipped triangle, in that before, she felt her risk was at the very bottom, the widest part of the triangle but that now, her risk was just at this tiny little peak of it. She was pleased by having reduced it to where she felt like she could live with the risk.

Like I said, what I wished more than anything was that they could say it's over. You never have to think about this again. There is zero risk. They were very clear in saying that a risk still remained, but that it is a diminished risk. Again, I just feel lucky that I've had a chance to do it this way and not in a crisis sort of situation. . . . I still check myself. I go over the surface of my skin and make sure I don't feel anything. I go under my armpits. I continue to go to the doctor and get checked. I know that there's still a small risk, but it's manageable. [Sandra]

That's life. I could die of colon cancer, too. I guess because it's such a small risk, relative to where I was, that I don't even think about it. I have much less risk of breast cancer than the average woman walking down the street, so what am I complaining about, even though there is a residual risk. [Joyce]

But, you know, if I get it, I don't know, it doesn't keep me awake at night at all. Somehow I have the sense that I won't get it, although I know that's foolish to be that relaxed about it. But I look at it as if, if I do get it—the thing about my mother was that no one could understand how she got it when I was five and it recurred when I was fourteen and she still lived until I was twenty-one. I knew she did because she was waiting for her youngest kid to be twenty-one. She just did everything. She tried every experimental thing. She did every test. She was a very good patient, and she did everything she could to fight it. The way I look at it, for what I have available today, then doing what I did is kind of like I did everything I could do to fight it. If I still get it, then that's what was meant to be. Then I would have had this operation anyway. . . . So if I'm going to have the operation anyway, I might as well have it at an early enough point that maybe it can really work because you can still have mastectomies and it could still have metastasized. So, I don't know. I mean if I still get, of course, I'm not going to love having it, but if I end up dying from it, I think that I still have it in my head that I gave it my best shot. That's all you can do really. It may be that I'll find out ten years from now I have some other horrible disease, you never know, you know. [Meredith]

NIPPLE SPARING

The issue in consideration of residual risk is how much breast tissue is left in surgery. There have been several waves of belief about this in the medical community. Early on, it was not widely recognized that sparing the nipple which can, in some cases, retain sensation, compromised the cancer prevention goal of the mastectomy. Later, there were strong feelings expressed in the medical community that the nipple should be completely removed to reduce to an absolute minimum the chances of the development of breast cancer. More recently, some authors have expressed the view that the risk of sparing the nipple is not so great at least in some well-defined circumstances.[3, 4] An interesting question is whether more lives would be saved overall by nipple sparing mastectomy, since it might induce more women to consider PM if nipple sensation could be retained. Two women here illustrate the weight of worry about residual nipple tissue.

> Yes [aware of residual risk]. In fact that was instilled enough so that they wouldn't let me keep my nipples, because in order to make sure that all the breast tissue was off, they'd have to scrape the nipple and, in turn, they wouldn't know whether they'd live or not. So they made it—they stressed the point that the possibility was still there. They had to take absolutely as much as they possibly could. Yes, I was aware of that.
> [How do you cope with the residual risk?] I forget it. [Ingrid]

> But the fact that I do have that breast tissue makes me feel as though I still have risk of developing cancer in the tissue that's existing. Well, just that the tissue that I had always has the potential to develop into cancerous tissue. I thought I would eliminate that by having a mastectomy. Now after that, I learned that all the tissue was not gone. So it's—but my percentage, and I've been told this, which makes me feel better, was reduced by 80 percent. So that's a little bit more comforting than if I had never had surgery. . . . Well, this is more because they did not take around the nipple, the areola, and they weren't sure they were going to, when going into the surgery, because they weren't sure if there was any other type of tissue any place else or if there was any more of the atypical hyperplasia. So they— They left it [the extra breast tissue]. I said, "I'd rather not." They were going to, and I said, "If you don't have to, please don't" because I thought that would be too disfiguring. They said, "Well, we'll make the decision last minute, and you really won't know until after the surgery." As it turned out, they did not take those areas. That's probably where the most concentration of tissue is left.

That tissue was also—I mean, that is tissue that can develop
cancer as well. That was a pretty good percentage at the time.
Also, that the tissue—the tissue left, it would be very superficial,
so things would be more visible.

Well, I do think about it in terms of I'm pretty healthy otherwise. I mean, I have a couple of other problems that—it hopefully
couldn't be fatal. I get migraines, although I know with my having migraines, the increase of stroke is higher. I don't smoke,
I don't drink. I'm pretty healthy physically. I'm not overweight.
In fact, depending on the time of year, I'm underweight sometimes. I don't get involved in any high-risk activities, so I think
that if that—if that is a risk that I have, that might be, outside of
an accident, that might be how I die, that will eventually come.
I maybe just bought some time. Maybe I would have bought
twenty years, twenty-five years by having surgery. So I do think
about that a lot. [Valerie].

FEELING DIFFERENT DOES NOT MEAN ONE
CANNOT FEEL GOOD

Adjustment after a prophylactic mastectomy takes many forms.
Some women talk about grieving for their old bodies. Other women
reject that idea, but may still have difficult moments recognizing the
changes that have occurred.

Yes, I never allowed myself to, like, suddenly go, "Oh, my God,
what have I done?" I wouldn't go there. [There is] —a set of rules
a set of different values that you put on certain things, like,
"Wow, that's a cool-looking outfit. Wow, that's a different look,"
or "Gee, I got my hair dyed purple. That's neat." I was trying to
just look at my body, because I knew I was going to see something that was going to shock me. So I guess I just changed what
this was all about it, and it was about how weird it's going to look,
and how it's going to change over the month and watching the
changes happen, and that it was all going to be part of this discovery of, "How did they do this thing?" and not about, "Oh, my
God, my body isn't the same body anymore." I just didn't—I
didn't allow myself to go there. By saying that, I know it sounds
like, "Oh, were you majorly in some denial?" ... I had a college
friend of mine ask me—well, actually tell me that, "Oh, you

obviously were in terrible denial and still are." This was like three years after the fact. And, "You've got to go through the mourning period."

I said, "Well, I'm sorry; but I've changed the rules." [Laughter] "I'm not going to go through a mourning period. I haven't gone through a mourning period."

I will say that I did have a moment—I had one moment. It was about thirty seconds long in the shower when I—about two weeks later [after the PM], I was in the shower. I have a skinny little, tiny shower in my bedroom, and I kind of bumped into myself somehow or the other, and my breast wasn't there. I remember going, "Oh, wow," and then I started to cry. I cried for probably about thirty seconds, and then I sort of felt stupid. I just felt really foolish because I felt like, "What's the point? It isn't there anymore. Get over it. Get used to the new deal." That's just how I did it. That was the end of it.

What it was all about, I was so happy that I had gotten rid of my time bomb, that the rest didn't seem terribly important, and I wasn't going to let society tell me that I should. [Laughs]. . . .

I think of the breasts, they're different; but to me, they're my new breasts. But I don't feel anything bad or anything unless— I'm walking around, breathing, acting, doing, lifting, carrying, doing things. But if I think about it, like right now, talking about it, I can feel little involuntary contractions of those muscles. Because like if you go to pick something up or you use your arm a certain way, you'll get a contraction in your pectoral muscles that if you have breasts, you don't feel it because those muscles aren't stretched out under your breasts. But mine are stretched out over an implant. So they're very taut anyway; but certain normal contractions for your chest muscles, you really feel them. They don't hurt; they just feel weird. [Fay]

It was a great. I went from a stinking little A cup to a D cup. I know. That's not what I'm supposed to say, right? Hey, hey, plenty of women pay a fortune for that, right? . . . I had said to Dr. X, "You know, I forget that they're not mine." They are mine, bought and paid for, but I forget that they aren't natural. They move with me. Everything about them feels natural. Of course, you don't have the feeling that's you—because it's just not there. [Ingrid]

That's strange [adjusting to new breasts]. I was always quite small. In fact, I was telling him, "I'm not looking for big breasts."

I just wanted to have a comfortable look so that I could wear clothes. I said, "If you gave me an A or a B cup, I'm fine. I'm not looking for anything any bigger." But it is bigger than what I was used to, and that sometimes feels strange. . . . I don't think that it's really affected it at all [sexual attractiveness], except for the uncomfortable feelings when I bend in certain ways. [Laura].

You still feel a little bit abnormal, but like I said, when you put your bra on, you get dressed, you can kind of forget about it. You can feel normal. But there are times when you feel a little bit, I guess, abnormal would be the right word and a little bit, yes, you feel a little bit strange. [Harriet]

It felt good, but it wasn't the real thing [having new breasts]. You felt differently knowing when you put your clothes on that it was something that would hold something. With the bra, you still felt that you're part of the female world. Do you know what I mean? It just kind of made you feel like you had something. That's how I felt. Nobody knows you have it. [Janice]

There are definite feelings of being changed that all of the women experienced after the prophylactic mastectomy. Some find positives in that change, but this rarely occurs without some feelings of unease or strangeness as women found their center again following surgery.

I was very small-breasted and I had two children. After many months of breastfeeding, there wasn't a lot of tissue there. There wasn't a lot of feeling in my nipples anymore because of that. Now I am a full [laughter] . . . To me this is busty. I have a 34A. So at first I felt like everybody would be staring at me because all of a sudden this is how I look. That's ridiculous now, but at the time that's how I felt, very much like I had just breast augmentation, which I did, but it was just so different for me to have that much cleavage after all that breastfeeding, so I felt very self-conscious for a very long time. I kept wearing big sweaters to hide it. . . . Yes, yes, because I had no idea what it would look like. It didn't look that bad at all . . . No. I don't feel like I had to adjust. No. I was more concerned with healing the scars and that kind of thing.

But I have to tell you, I personally look better in clothes, so that part wasn't an adjustment at all. That was kind of a surprise. I didn't think that would be any big deal to me, but it was actually a nice surprise. Great. I feel like it's no longer this thing that's going to bail on me or betray me. It's an odd thing to think about your body, but I don't feel that about it anymore. I look terrific. In fact, my friends who I have told them about this, tease me because I shouldn't look this good as a forty-year-old woman with two children. [unclear] They kind of friendly tease me about it, but physically he [the plastic surgeon] did a really good job. In fact, I don't have very large scars at all anymore. In fact, they almost look like just stretch marks kind of things. Physically, there's no—sometimes I feel a little like if I'm doing something with both hands out in front of me, I feel a little loss of muscle. But it's so slight that it's really not even. Even how the muscles are all stretched around, I can understand how that should be. But it's nothing that ever hurts or is uncomfortable or anything like that. It's an odd sort of feeling that you get used to. [Kate]

HOW LONG TO FEEL NORMAL AGAIN?

When embarking on any surgery, but especially one as complex as the process of surgically altering one's breasts, it is evident that both the surgery and recovery will be "front-burner" concerns for the immediate future. A woman needs to take leave from work, to arrange childcare, to have help physically for self-care, meals, etc. for the period of hospitalization and recovery from surgery. Physicians can estimate how long this period is likely to be, so a woman typically has a sense of how long she will be officially "out of commission" as a result of the surgery.

But how long does it take to actually feel like oneself, to not be thinking about the surgery and its impact? Is there a postsurgery "normal" experience? This is a question best answered by women who have had a bilateral PM. While new surgical techniques in the future may alter the pace of recovery, it is clear from women's responses that feeling normal is psychological in nature, and is tied to, but not identical with, recovering function and feeling.

There was enormous variation in how women responded to the question of how long it took for them to get back to normal. We did not define "normal" and, hence, what the women meant by normal was their own configuration. It is also clear that this is a "new normal," and that there are unpleasant reminders of the surgery even long after the woman is generally back doing most normal activities. Perhaps, the range is best illustrated just by listing here the responses women gave to this important question.

Well, it came back to normal, I don't know what you call normal. I don't know. That's a hard question to answer, because I don't think—I don't know how to answer that. Oh, physically, well, you never feel the same. I would say about 20 percent of my chest area is still numb. When you wear the bra, it hurts. [Kristen]

It's hard to remember really. You never get back to normal normal, you know, because it's, you know, but, you know, it got back to pretty normal pretty fast, I guess. I mean, this isn't normal, too. Right, it's not normal ... But, yes, I'd say I adjusted, you know, probably, well, very fast. [Alice]

A month really for me was the major—that was the major chunk of recovery time for me. Meaning that after a month, I went to Disney World and went on every ride, and I wasn't feeling 100 percent, but I was able to do a lot of stuff and get tossed around and go on roller coasters and do thing. It kind of hurt a little. I was just getting back to myself ... [So it took about a month to feel back to normal?] Yes. I don't work a regular job. ...

But I felt weak, and I felt—and one thing I noticed because I'm a singer, I was supposed to do a concert about—I forget, maybe—it was in March, and I had the surgery in January. In February, I started trying to prepare for this concert. I sang with an orchestra and I couldn't get my breath. I mean, I couldn't get through two words of the song without feeling totally winded, much less have the air [unclear] to produce the sounds that I needed to produce. So that took me—again, it took me a few months to just get my kind of lung-power back. I don't know if it's because it hurts because of the muscles were sore. You know, because your muscles were stretching out, and everything has been kind of disturbed in that area of your body that there was soreness. [Fay]

That's 100 percent normal, 100 percent normal. It was right away. I mean, since I was healed, I got back into work, and the kids activities and coming and going and moving ... I'd say, to have it perfectly back to normal, probably about three weeks. [Chantal]

Well, the only area that it didn't come back to normal was my physical health, my endurance, my stamina. Everything else, probably after about—it took about four months and it was mostly because of the sensations, it gradually, gradually went away. I thought they would never go away. But maybe about four, five months. [Valerie]

I thought I would be down and out for months. But I was up and running, I think, well, he took my drains out. I begged Dr. X to take my drains out. . . . I think it took me two weeks, and I was ready. I'd say within three months here. Again, it depends on where you are in your life. I happen to be in—three years later, I had a baby. [Beth]

Oh, I would say, well, for me, I mean I think part of it is going through the reconstruction and all of that. So, depending on all of that. But, it's been just over a year for me now, and I mean I think I can securely say that I feel like things are normal now. I went through a period even with my implants where I felt like, oh, these things are hard as rock, should I have done this, dah, dah, dah, dah, dah. It took several months, but I feel like they have finally softened up now and are much more normal, and I'm comfortable with them. I sleep all right. I'd say a year. [Irene]

I was moving around pretty well within a week. I find that my life was normal within not very long. By that, I'm going to say, by the time, within a couple of months. I mean it's not a hundred percent normal, because things are not over with. [Sonia]

I actually went home from the hospital a day sooner than I was supposed to . . . And I just kept visualizing that and six weeks down the road I was still sort of human again. Still it is, it's a three month, if you do TRAM flap, it's a good three months of recovery, and it's really a year before you really feel good again. You're tired for a year . . . I'm a bartender, so I'm juggling working at night and then getting up four hours later to get my kids off to school. Then my little one is only a half day, so then I go back to bed for like two hours and get [up] again to get him.

You know how it is, when you're working so much that you're just so busy that if you do have problems you just don't have that much time to dwell on it . . . I find that now, anyway. I think it's just something to do with being forty-two or the winter or something. But it took a good three months to feel . . . I didn't get back to work for four months because my job is very physical. It took a good three months to feel like I'd go out with my friends and go do things normally and get into a normal workout schedule and be able to do all my housework again and take care of my kids without any extra help once in a while. [Meredith]

Twelve weeks. I think as soon as you get a normal prosthesis. Probably, I'd say 12 weeks is a good—you feel you're doing everything, and I think the body image, or at least for me, will last a lifetime. [Julia]

One to one and half years. I'd say about a year, about a year and a half. Basically, after my depression left, I felt like life got to be normal. I guess I felt really good. [Hanna]

Let me think. Maybe a year. [Laura]

Six months. It took a while [to feel normal again], because I think they were afraid I was going to break or afraid that I was going to do something, but it took about like maybe a good six months. I was healing and feeling happy and getting back to work. Once I started getting back to work and getting into a routine, I think that kind of let them know that everything was okay. [Janice]

Presurgery. When I made the decision to have the surgery. [Vicky]

Six months. I didn't realize how much it was affecting me until about six months after the surgery. My life was back to normal. Yes, better than. What's normal? It was better than normal. [Joyce]

Seven months. Yes, I think everything was back pretty much to normal, and probably, like I say, I was out of work for seven months because I stayed out right through until even I had the nipples reconstructed and everything before I went back to work. So pretty much about by the time I went back to work, things were pretty much back to normal. [Emily]

I have to say it took a couple of months to really feel like I could do more. It took, I would say, a year until I really felt totally normal. . . . As I said earlier, physically, I felt a year. I think really longer than that sort of psychologically. I really do feel that I have that now, whereas I said some things, I am annoyed that I can't go to the locker room the same way and things. I have new limitations, there's no doubt. So, it's not a hundred percent normal. [Sandra]

About four to six weeks I felt like I was right back to normal. Very quickly. I had an incredible sense of triumph and relief that the whole process was over. [Rose]

These different assessments of the time it took for the return to normalcy contain all of the continuing challenge and the triumph which a prophylactic mastectomy seems to leave women with. Life is changed in many ways and the recovery is definitely both physical and emotional. We will hear more in subsequent chapters about how women perceived the changes in themselves and in their relationships to others.

CHAPTER 6

Sex and Sensitivity after Surgery

Breasts serve many functions during a woman's life. For adult women, breasts are a source of sexual pleasure and arousal as well as a means of attracting and arousing a sexual partner. A significant worry for a woman undergoing mastectomy, either for cancer or prophylactically, is whether she will be less attractive sexually after surgery and, as a result of the loss of breast and nipple sensation and diminished self-image, less sexually responsive. Most women who consider prophylactic mastectomy (PM) do so only after they have long established marriages or partnerships. Relatively few single, young woman have undergone PM, though this may be changing as second generation young women become aware earlier of their mutation status. For women at high hereditary risk of breast cancer due to *BRCA1/2* or other mutations, breast cancer can occur earlier than for women in the general population. Thus, women at hereditary risk in their 40s or 30s and, even occasionally, in their 20s may undergo prophylactic mastectomy. Prophylactic mastectomy occurs, then, at a time when sexual functioning is of major importance to the woman and to her sexual partner. Even for women in their 50s or 60s, sexual attraction and functioning are important in their assessment of the costs and benefits of PM. Understandably, much of a woman's concern about the outcomes of PM center on how attractive she thinks she will feel, how attractive she will be to her mate or partners, and to what degree the surgery will interfere with their sexual pleasure and emotional relationship.

The women we interviewed were remarkably candid about their postsurgery sense of their bodies and the impact of PM on their intimate relationships. Some even asked if they were telling us more than we wanted to know, which, of course, was not the case. While the candor is a tribute to the trust developed during the interview, it may also be that this crucially important issue for many women is one which they feel they cannot truly discuss with many friends and, often, not even with their spouses or partners. The private or "taboo" aspect may have contributed to their willingness to share their views, especially in the relative safety of a telephone interview.

A core issue is the question of how central breasts are to a particular woman's sense of herself and, here, not surprisingly the range of answers was quite broad. While some women were adamant that breasts do not make a woman, other women clearly had markedly increased sexual insecurity about how attractive they were after surgery to their husbands or, if not partnered, to others, generally.

Sexual impact and adjustment had much to do with the woman's sense of postsurgical "normalcy." Along with concern about the impact of PM surgery, there were also interesting interjections of more usual worries women had about their weight or about the impact of aging on their bodies, their self-esteem, and self-image. This helped to provide a yardstick against which some women measured the impact of surgery.

WHERE IS MY FEMININITY?

Sonia told us, "It's in my mind [my femininity]. It's in myself. It's who I am. Not my boobs." Most women agreed that not having breasts did not eradicate their femininity or even vastly change their own feelings about their femininity, but the extent to which women felt that others would feel similarly differed greatly. Even internally, some women contrasted their own strongly held beliefs that breasts were not essential to being a woman with their experience, especially early after surgery, that they felt less womanly.

But the reason I say a year is by then our body really has healed and you've worked through it and your arms are moving and you're sitting up and laying and doing the things that you're used to. That's when I found I had the worst, because it was like it hit me. I just did not feel like I was a woman anymore. I felt like I was just in a woman's body, but I wasn't whole. I'm know I'm whole, but at that time you could tell me I was whole, but I'd say, "No,

I'm not," because I didn't have breasts. But breasts is [sic] not what makes a woman. [Hanna]

This clearly is a difficult conundrum for these conflicted women. Intellectually, they understand that breasts are only a part of a woman's attractiveness and responsiveness, and that, after the breasts are removed, they can remain active, sexual, attractive women without breasts. Emotionally, however, their deep feelings belie this knowledge and they believe they are lacking an essential element in their sexual attractiveness and that even a longtime partner may not find them as attractive or even attractive. From our interviews, it is apparent, that such negative feelings often persist even when spouses are verbally supportive and clear about their continuing, sexual interest.

We speculate that it may be that some of the difficulty comes from the lack of open, honest discussion in many of the couples about the losses associated with mastectomy. It is true that mastectomy leads to the loss of a source of pleasure for both partners. As the narratives in this chapter attest to, many women felt a deep sense of loss with the surgical removal of their breasts. Only a few talked about having discussed with their partner about what this might feel like before surgery or what it did mean after surgery. The openness of the women in talking to us, the depth of their sense of loss, even those with very positive outcomes and supportive partners, and the rarity of reports about joint spousal discussions, either before or after surgery, about the physical losses and changes mastectomy would bring to their sexual lives suggest that it might be helpful for couples to be encouraged and guided to talk more openly before PM surgery. There seemed to be in many cases, a strong and immediate need for partners to only reassure the woman, to only talk about the positives, to say clearly that the relationship, sexual and otherwise, would overcome the surgical changes and continue to be satisfying, perhaps even more satisfying because of diminished fears about breast cancer disrupting their lives. However, honest talk might actually itself be prophylactic, at least in marriages or relationships where open communication is the norm for other sensitive topics.

NOT A BIG DEAL

A few women played down the importance of breasts and, thus, the significance of having them removed.

I don't know how to explain it to you because it's funny. Breasts are an appendage, and men make such a big deal out of them. I think women are made to feel like they are just an object anyway. So to remove them and put something in there that looks just as good or almost as good is not a big deal. [Meredith]

[How was it emotionally to adjust to new breasts?] Nothing. It wasn't one way or the other. I honestly can say nothing, no big deal to me. I could have gone with nothing. I don't have a problem with, "Oh, I don't have breasts, I can't be looking over there." Doesn't bother me. [Vicky]

AM I STILL ATTRACTIVE?–HOW I FEEL

Sex did not come as naturally to some women after PM. There were adjustments to make. Sensation was less available and worry about attractiveness hampered spontaneous enjoyment. Harriet said her interest and enjoyment were not less than presurgery, but that she was less sexually responsive which she attributed to her own evaluation of her attractiveness.

Not interest and enjoyment, no, but as far as how you feel about yourself, you have to really like make a conscious effort . . . to try to feel attractive, to try to feel okay with yourself. You have to work on it, whereas before, it came. It's the natural thing for a woman . . . I find myself like forcing myself to feel attractive. [Harriet]

The openness of the women we interviewed extended to telling us things they clearly wished they were not feeling or had not felt about their attractiveness or about their bodies.

Oh, yes, I don't feel sexually attractive, but I don't feel sexually unattractive. My biggest fear is, this sounds silly, you know, my husband was in (a foreign city) for business and I was panicked. He's never gone there before. I said, "Oh, my God, you take care of yourself, you go to the hotel." In the back of my mind is, "If anything ever happened to him, I'd probably never have a relationship again." Now, most women don't think that. They think they'd miss their husband. I'm thinking nobody would ever want to love me because I don't have breasts. I do feel that . . . My husband once made, . . . because I talked to him about it, and he said, "That's terrible. People would love you." He says, "You're a great person." He said, "You can still have a relationship" ... we'd have very in-depth talks, and that's why I feel I'm very fortunate. But, I always would turn whatever he said kind of negative, because I guess I really don't feel great about my femininity. I don't, but life goes on. Nothing's perfect, you know. [Julia]

The strength of this woman's self-doubt about her attractiveness was further underscored in a conversation she had with friends. She said:

If I make some remarks about my husband, you know, if you're talking, and I'll go, "Oh, I've got to be good to [him]," I said, "because, you know, he could stray real easy with what I have to offer." ... They go, "Oh, stop that." They'll cut me off. I go, "What, I do worry about it." I said, "I certainly don't have a chest to offer. It's not at all sexually attractive." They'll just say, "Stop it." It's only because they don't know what to say and because I say it so tongue-in-cheekish. But I really do feel like that.

Another woman had, she says, made her peace with her body being changed, and it led her to alter her behavior in certain ways.

I feel like they're just a thing. They are not really my new breasts. I am adamant about that, they're not my new breasts. Your breasts are gone and I was in touch with that process and I was able to let my breasts go ... I'm hard with myself. But now what it is, I shop more than usual. I look fine. I forget about it. What's interesting about my breasts now is that they don't have feelings, they feel different. I can see in my body when I have goose bumps where the goose bumps stop, and I hold back from hugging people because I don't like the way my breasts feel. They feel like they're rock solid. Like I'm hugging a basketball. [Rose]

Sandra's comments about her "Barbie breasts" conveyed her discomfort and sense of distance from seeing herself as a grown woman:

Because of my reconstruction [I feel uncomfortable]. I didn't do the nipples. So, I look like I have Barbie breasts, the tan bumps with nothing on them.

IS SEX DIFFERENT? INTERACTION
WITH THE PARTNER

Some women responded to questions about their sexual experience
and the impact of PM by talking mainly about themselves while others
couched their answers in terms of the impact on their husbands or
partners.

No, because they were never a real source of pleasure to me in the
first place. I wouldn't say it really affected him, because he, how
do I put it, he wasn't that—how can I say it—he's not a breast
man. No, my breasts were not really the sexual issue for us. Well,
for a while there, he thought he was going to hurt me if he
touched me. [Kristen]
     My husband, I didn't let him see me right after the surgery for
a while. I didn't want him to have detailed memories of me like
that. [Rose]

Hanna spoke of the time after "we" had the PM surgery as being
difficult.

Somewhat, a little, a little [loss of sexual attractiveness]. It doesn't
hold the whole thing. I know that if my husband, because he
doesn't say it because he's not like that. I feel that it would be a
little different, because we were married for a long time before
we had it done. I know that after we had the surgery, he was pet-
rified to touch me. He had things that he had to work through,
too, and it took a long time before he could touch me. [How long
did it take?] Almost a year. And that was hard on me because I felt
like, "What have I done?" That was hard.

Meredith, unlike most women who talked about missing sensation
in her nipples, talked about some retained or phantom feeling there.
This phenomenon has been reported in the medical literature.[1]

But the weird part, I don't know how to explain it, is that even
though I don't really have a lot of feeling, like if—and it's
improved. I guess because it's my own tissue and there is something called re-enervation. Like in the beginning, if you took an
ice cold can of soda and you put it on my breast, I couldn't tell.
Now I can sort of feel that it's cold. When we're having sex and

he does things to my nipples, I still can feel it as if I still had it. I think it's like a phantom, because my brain knows that I should be feeling. So when we're doing things sexually, and he plays with my nipples, I can still feel it.

The other weird thing is that when I'm in public and a baby cries, I still get the tingling and the [unclear] feeling. It's like if you cut off your arm and people have that phantom arm thing. I'm having a phantom breast thing. So in that way, it's not a bad thing, because when you're actually in the middle of having sex, and like I said, my husband really never noticed. I mean if he noticed he was real good at not showing it, because he says he'd rather have me alive. In fact he didn't even care if I had the reconstruction. [Meredith]

Women did speak of the loss of nipple and breast sensation as something which affected them and sometimes their spouses significantly. They also talked about accommodation in their sexual practices to work around this loss of an erogenous zone.

I feel because of the way—first of all, sex isn't the same . . . I still enjoy sex a whole lot, and so does he. I wouldn't say we have problems or anything. But it's definitely changed. I mean, there was feeling in that area and, you know, that's gone. So we've given up that, to have, you know. It's not what it was, so that's definitely giving up there. Plus, with all of the society's images of what a beautiful woman is, I mean, he has never done anything, except I feel like he's given it up. I mean, you know . . . The only thing, the changes are what had to be, you know? It's not like I was more up tight, just in my own head. It's just something we had to go through because of the circumstances. So, you know, and I feel the loss, I do feel the loss. [Alice]

We're still in a very healthy sex life . . . We've always had a very good relationship. I would not recommend this for a couple whose relationship is based strictly on attraction and sex, because you are different; you no longer have breasts, and if your husband was a breast man, you're in trouble. So, you know, I think that before a couple does it, they really need to talk about it and the changes and —I mean, I still can have children and there's bottles that you can feed them with, so it doesn't prohibit you from having family. But there has to be a strong—there has to be a basis to your relationship other than sex and physical attraction . . . No, I mean, it's just you have to be—you both have to be positive about it. It's not something to jump into and, you know, it's something to talk about and be open about it, and, you know, it's okay. You both can mourn the loss of it if you want, but you still can enjoy life. We have a great relationship still, and—you know, it hasn't changed anything. [Chantal]

You definitely miss the part. I'm not going to tell you, I mean, you definitely, it's not like there's something not missing. There's something definitely missing . . . Just that there's no feeling anymore, and they're not squishy . . . It's one thing that's pretty much the same. I think you just kind of—I don't want to get graphic, but I think you do different things . . . You just get better about it. Look-wise, they look great. They look much better than normal ones. But feel-wise, it's not there. There's no feeling. [Beth]

It's funny. The breasts didn't bother me, but I miss the nipples. The nipples, well, first of all, you don't have any nipples for like nine months. Nipples, well, they say, they are for kids, well, yes, they are. You nurse your kids with them and they do things when you're having sex. Fake nipples don't do that. They don't have much feeling, and they're not the same. So, I find I have nipple envy. I picture the women who have nipples. Like real breasts are more torpedo shaped. Mine are more round. It's hard to find a bra that actually fits them right and that kind of thing . . . But the nipples aren't real, and they don't do the things real nipples do. I don't know. So I don't miss my breasts that much, but I miss my nipples. [Meredith]

Other women whom we interviewed for the study felt that the impact of the PM surgery on their spouses was minimal.

With clothes off, yes [it does affect my sense of sexual attractiveness]. Again, because they don't move naturally so it's just—it looks awkward. Even though it doesn't—I know you're going to ask me about my husband, but it doesn't make any difference to him; it does to me. [Valerie]

Well, it certainly, I mean with losing, I certainly have lost the sensation that I had in my breasts before. So, from a sexual standpoint, that's definitely changed because I don't. I can feel it if somebody touches my breasts, if my husband touches my breast, but I don't have that same sexual stimulation that I might have had before. So, I definitely have lost that . . . I think initially I had some concerns about that [change in sex interests], but my husband is so pleased with the reconstruction that it certainly hasn't affected his interest. And, so, that, in turn, I think, makes me feel good about myself and helps me. So, I would say, overall, it hasn't had any real noticeable impact. [Irene]

SOME THINGS ARE BETTER, BUT STILL A LOSS

Displeasure with one's previous breast shape would seemingly have made it easier for some women to accept the idea of PM and to find the results to be pleasing. However, Sandra talked about the fact that her sense of the improvement in body shape postsurgery did not diminish the sense of loss she experienced about changes in her body shape, no matter how unhappy she had been about it.

I think all of us have different relationships with our breasts. I think it might be difficult for somebody who really felt very, very positively about her breasts, that they are very beautiful parts of her body. I didn't really. I always felt that they were just too big for my body. There was a slight embarrassment about having D cups, so, oddly enough that sort of played in my favor in making it less of a loss than it might have been. So, when I did the surgery, I asked for B cups, and there was a little improvement on the whole ... I don't mean to minimize, but there is still loss. You're losing your breast, you're losing an extremely important part of who you are and your sexuality. So, I don't mean to minimize that. But there were some pluses in that, I mean, I even still feel that today. I'm always happy ... Yes, I mean there was definitely sort of a loss, even though, as I said, I wasn't crazy about my breasts, they were my breasts. They had, you know, they were part of who I was as a sexual being, and that was a real adjustment. I mean that was a real loss. There is no doubt about that. [Sandra]

HUMOR AND SELF-IMAGE

While feelings of loss did not engender regret about the PM surgery, which was almost always viewed as having been a good decision, they were powerful. Sometimes humor was called upon to cope with the mixture of emotions women reported.

Yes, I never allowed myself to, like, suddenly go, "Oh, my God, what have I done?" I wouldn't go there I was very—I was very

attached to my old breasts. They had names. I think they were—
Sam and Irving. [Fay]

Joking about the rearranged parts of their body which had been
used to make their new breasts helped some women and their sexual
partners to find lightness in the adjustment to differentness. Ingrid
told us:

> So that's the way we had to make light of some of the situations.
> I had the cartilage removed from the back of my ear to put in
> the nipple, so I used to say, "You've got to come closer, I can't
> hear you. [Ingrid]
>   No different, I don't think. I think my husband may have
> another question, because he keeps making a joke of me being a
> Picasso now, because my stomach's now up in my chest. We have
> inside jokes, but it's fine. He doesn't have a problem with it at all.
> Neither do I. [Vicky]

REFLECTED POSITIVE AESTHETICS

As is also true for women who have not had PM, for some women it
is how others perceive them that largely determines how they feel
about their bodies. In one woman's story, it was the surgeon's
judgment, as relayed by recovery room nurses that enhanced her sense
of satisfaction.

> [After] I went back in for the final implants to be put in, a couple
> of things happened that I think were very positive that might not
> happen to all women. But the nurse who was in the recovery
> room came up to me after the surgery, and she said, "You know,
> we were talking about your breast reconstruction over lunch."
> She said, "We were saying what a nice job Dr. X does, and, in
> particular, we were saying what a nice job he did with you." To
> have somebody tell you that when you're in the recovery room
> was a real booster for me. The idea that these nurses were sitting
> around lunch talking about how good my boobs looked was—and
> I don't think that they do that to everybody, but he did really
> build me a very nice set, and the nurses were talking about it over
> lunch. So right away I felt really good about it, and then I've done
> nothing but feel positive about it ever since because he looked at

them and he said, "They're the best that I've ever done." This is a lot of positive reinforcement coming back. I'm sure he doesn't say that to everybody. I told him he could have a picture if he wanted to. [Joyce].

FEELING CLOSER TOGETHER

For some couples, postsurgical intimacy and closeness generally was said to be enhanced.

Has it changed anything there [with intimacy]? I think because I feel so much better about myself, maybe, and my body, that maybe I'm enjoying it more. But the difference is probably very slight. I don't think that's changed. I look fabulous, so there's no ugly scarring or anything like that. Just that I feel so good about it, which was just the surprising thing, too. [Kate]

Also, I did have a certain sense of worry that he would miss my old breasts. But he always reassures me that that doesn't bother him at all . . . I will say that having gone through the whole surgery thing and the whole experience, that if anything, I think it made my husband appreciate me, love me, and respect me even more because he thought it took an amazing amount of bravado and courage or whatever to go through all this. Whereas I laugh at that because I always say, "It wasn't really bravado. I was doing what I felt—it was pragmatic thing." [Fay]

DATING (SINGLE AT THE TIME)

Sandra was remarried at the time of the interview, although she had had a prior period of being single postsurgery when dating and sexuality had been challenging.

[How was dating?] That was very hard. I really, as I said, I dated one person, and I felt really uncomfortable even broaching that. I did finally tell him. He was really shocked. Shocked, but sort of supportive, but really visibly shocked at the thought. I do remember [telling my date about the PM]. I remember saying, "I have to tell you something." I really had a hard time saying it. He was like, "What, what, what, what is it, what is it?" He was really becoming alarmed. He was really not imagining at all what it was. I don't think anybody would jump to that possible conclusion. [I remember] him being very surprised. I think it was somebody I had just dated three or four months, and obviously going very slowly, it's just my feeling that you do have to go very slowly in this sort of situation. I mean I think for other reasons, we just—it didn't go any further . . .

I would say no [I don't feel less attractive], but I think I feel that I didn't feel great about them before, and now I feel, because of the relationship I'm in, totally appreciated and feel very, very comfortable with that, and with how my breasts are looked at, and how they play into the relationship is very positive . . . . Well, first of all, I was convinced there was no man in the world who would look at me, based on the fact that I had mastectomies. If I had just had implants with my regular tissue, then that would be different; but I thought I was too disfigured to be attractive to anybody else. Not that I even wanted to be attractive to my ex-husband. That wasn't an issue for me. I thought it would be a huge challenge for me to get anybody interested in me based on my physical appearance. . . . With clothes off, yes [it does affect my sense of sexual attractiveness]. Again, because they don't move naturally so it's just—it looks awkward . . . I know you're going to ask me about my husband, but it doesn't make any difference to him; it does to me. No, not really [didn't affect my interest in sex]. There really hasn't been any change. I think the change happened I had more interest after I remarried.

INTEGRATING AND ADJUSTING

Time is clearly an important factor in women's postsurgery adjustment. It takes a while to recover from the physical insults of surgery and to change one's clothing as needed and to stop having thoughts about PM surgery on the "front burner." But how long it takes to get to feeling that thinking about surgery has come to be "back burner" will vary.

I remember it was about a year and a half later when my husband and I were at a party, a going-away party for one of his managers, and one of his bosses had come up to me and he had started to tell me how pretty he thought I was and all this and that. I couldn't figure out what he was talking about. Then I realized and I think he realized, and he said, "Oh, I'm so sorry." I'm like, "It's no big deal. I don't mind." But I said to him, "Actually, it's kind of refreshing, because I think it's the first time in a long time that I'd actually even forgotten I'd done it." To a point where it's almost that I have to remember that I did it. [Meredith]

The topic of PM surgery seems to break down certain social norms. When women are open about their impending or recent surgery, it focuses attention, including visual attention, on their breasts. Breasts become "social property," much the way people feel free to pat the stomachs of pregnant women or comment on their weight gain. Women told us that postsurgery they were aware that others would immediately look at their chests out of curiosity to see if they could detect the changes in the shape of their breasts. As we have mentioned, some women also showed their breasts to friends or colleagues post-surgery, something they would not have done previously. Meredith talked about her husband's boss commenting favorably on her appearance. She was not taken aback by this conversation as a flirtatious gesture; rather, she saw it as the boss's way of making a positive comment on her postsurgical status, a comment which made her realize how far she had come in putting thoughts about the appearance of her breasts on the "back burner."

Valerie also spoke of adjusting to the comments and glances of others.

To myself, they [my breasts] were noticeable with me. I could—I got used to them faster than everybody else got looking at me. So that—I mean, I never boasted about having larger breasts after my surgery. I certainly—I don't want them or anything, but just the people who knew me noticed a difference. So it was kind of a little bit uncomfortable, having people look just out of curiosity. Then when they say things like, "Oh, gee, well, you can't even tell," and you know that they've actually been looking.

I never—I was never one to bring attention to any part of my body. The breasts is [sic] not a woman—it's where guys always look and now I have everybody looking. So it was quite a bit of adjustment. I guess I have told everybody that I knew practically that this was happening to me. I mean, how can I expect them not to look? So I'm thinking in terms of what if I haven't said anything to anybody, what would they think? Maybe I was just

wearing a pushup bra or something, a padded bra. They certainly
wouldn't make a point of looking and then commenting. [Valerie]

CLOTHING AND BRAS

The physical changes which PM brings mean that clothes do not fit
in the same way they did before. For some women, this was freeing;
some who have elected not to have breast reconstruction enjoyed feeling they did not have to worry about wearing a bra. For others, there
was more of an adjustment.

I spoke to her [woman who had previously undergone PM] about
it and she said, "You know, one of the great things is that you
don't have to wear a bra." I guess at the time I didn't appreciate
what it was she was talking about. Hey, you know, it's wonderful.
You don't have to wear a bra because your muscles hold your
boobs in place and that means you can throw on any little tank
top or anything and just go running out, and you look great. So
it's very comfortable because you're not confined. You don't realize how much those straps really are confining until you don't
have to wear them anymore. [Joyce]

This is kind of minor, but the only thing that seemed like
somewhat of an adjustment is, for the longest time I kept trying
to find a bra that was comfortable to fit, thinking I still needed
to wear a bra. Basically, I eventually ended up just giving up on
it. I don't need to wear a bra for support or anything because
the implants are self-supporting. I could never find a bra that
fit the shape of them right and was comfortable. That's the only
thing. I bought more bras thinking, "Oh, I'll try it on. This one's
going to be great." I'd wear it like one day and ditch it, get rid of
it. [Emily]

What was helpful? I mean when you go and get fitted for your
bras and this and that, you can feel semi back to a normal figure....
You still feel a little bit abnormal, but like I said, when you put your
bra on, you get dressed, you can kind of forget about it. You can
feel normal. But there are times when you feel a little bit, I guess,
abnormal would be the right word and a little bit, yes, you feel a little bit strange. [Harriet]

It felt good. It felt good, but it wasn't the real thing [having
new breasts]. You felt differently knowing when you put your

clothes on that it was something that would hold something. With the bra, you still felt that you're part of the female world. [Janice]

Other women seemed to have fewer issues about the fit of clothing; in one case, the woman felt it was not a concern because she had always had small breasts.

But it wasn't a big thing. Again, I think it comes down to, also, your size that you were. Like I said, I was very tiny to begin with. It really was not a—my clothes still fit the same. I never wear— they gave me those little padded . . . They stick in your T-shirt, and I never even wear them. [Chantal]

We just go to a party this last year, and I was wearing the slinkiest dress and I don't wear a bra. So, no, I don't have any problem with my body. [Sonia]

WEIGHT AND AGING CHANGES ONE'S BODY, TOO

Asking postmastectomy women how they felt about their bodies brought up issues other than the impact of mastectomy. Whether this was defensive or not, whether it was a distraction, or whether, indeed, weight or aging were just more charged (and possibly more long-standing) concerns related to body image for some women, these issues came into our interviews with some frequency.

[Currently feel about body?] Fine. A little heavy, but that's true of everybody in the world. [Vicky]

Probably the overweight, definitely the overweight part both-ers me more than the mastectomy part. I mean, I'm not real huge or anything, but—.[Alice]

Well, I wish I could lose about fifteen pounds, which I've gained since then, just because I'm in my forties now and my body is slowing down. But, as far as my breasts go, it's not that as much as, in general, I wish I had more time to work out and lose weight. [Meredith]

I hate my body anyway . . . Oh, gosh. An aging body. [Beth]

Interestingly, for Beth, the fact that her reconstructed breasts did not sag was what she found herself somewhat embarrassed about over

time. She felt this marked her has having something artificial, something which made her different from her contemporaries.

> Yes, I still haven't gotten over it. They're very stiff and very hard
> and very unmoving. I think, you know, it's funny, but the older I
> get, the more I know I should be sagging. The less I'm sagging,
> and the more I think it shows, as opposed to when seven years
> ago, when it just looked good . . . I just feel like they're awfully
> perky [for my age].

TO FEEL GRATEFUL

Overall, however, many women, while acknowledging losses and
needed adjustments related to loss of their breasts, spoke of their
enormous relief and gratitude that they could have prophylactic surgery to substantially reduce their risk for breast cancer.

> My feeling was, you know, I can live without breasts as long as I
> can live. I felt sort of fortunate to be given the choice, to have
> the option to decide in this way, and not to be in the place, pos-
> sibly a few years down the line, where I wouldn't have such a
> luxurious choice, in a sense. [Sandra]
> I feel great about myself, and I just basically hope that people
> don't stop doing it, because of, my God, this is my breasts, and
> my breasts is [sic] my femininity and all of that crap. If I had
> had that said to me, you've got to feel terrible. It's like, "No,
> I don't feel terrible. I feel great." [Sonia]

CHAPTER 7

In Sickness and in Health: Post-Surgical Relationship with Spouses, Partners and Others

POST-SURGICAL RELATIONSHIP WITH SPOUSES, AND PARTNERS AND OTHERS

Feeling Closer—or Not

Adversity can sometimes bring a couple together. While bilateral prophylactic mastectomy (PM) surgery is a major event in any marriage, how the couple handles it can result in the two people feeling closer or, especially for already vulnerable marriages, have the opposite effect. With the decision to have the surgery, the woman has taken a huge step towards safety and away from fear about breast cancer and its potentially deadly threat to her (and to the couple). What makes people feel close, how much they discuss or do not discuss the surgery, either before or after the procedure varies greatly. Not surprisingly, how surgery impacts the marriage or relationship is a function of the pre-existing relationship, but also of the sensitivities of each partner and how much the other person understands their partner's reasoning and responds in desired ways. Of the women in our study, there were very few who reported major negative effects of surgery on the important intimate relationship in their lives.

For many of the couples in our group, the issue of prophylactic mastectomy came up after they had spent many years together and weathered other crises (not infrequently including the breast cancer of other family members). Their sexual relationship was therefore well-established. For other couples, the issue of this surgery came up early in their years together and at the peak of their sexual relationship.

And for a small minority, the prospect of surgery predated their relationship and discussion of it came up early in their lives together, sometimes even predating their commitment.

In a troubled marriage, PM can lead to great misunderstanding, hurt feelings on either side, and may be a factor in the decision or timing to end the relationship. Problems can arise over a number of issues—whether the woman feels opposed in her decision; whether the man feels ignored or feels his opinion was unwanted or treated as irrelevant; whether the man accompanies his partner on medical visits; how the man acts during the woman's hospitalization; what kind of caregiver he is postsurgery when the woman returns home; whether there is an effort to provide a comfortable, accepting, postsurgical home; and how the couple deals with the physical changes that result. These problems can all have a big impact on a fragile marriage. This surgery is not occasioned by medical necessity, but rather is a choice, and, therefore, is more subject to interpretation and resentment by a partner who feels left out of the decision. It changes an axis of sexual pleasure for the couple, which, again, can arouse emotional sensitivities. It has the potential to become the fulcrum on which the marriage either improves or falters.

Our interviews were only with the women who had undergone PM; we do not truly have the partners' views first hand. The interview questions were focused on how the woman felt she and her partner had reacted to the surgery and its consequences. In Chapter 6, we have examined the woman's views of her partner's physical and emotional responses to the surgery in the intimate sphere of sex. In this chapter, we present the information gathered when we asked more about the full impact of the surgery on the entire relationship, if the relationship was changed at all and, if so, how and why.

Some women framed the discussions they had with their partners around their wish to undergo PM as a test, or, at least retrospectively, they looked at it that way. The test was of how the partner valued the woman's potentially increased longevity if the woman had a PM and how the partner weighed the physical versus the emotional aspects of their relationship.

My husband, I love and adore deeply, and he does me, as well. So I don't know what I would have done without him because he really supported me through this thing, so much that I'm forever indebted to him because he helped me through some bad times . . .

[Did surgery affect the quality of marriage?] No, because that's not my husband. My husband, like he had told me prior, breasts are breasts. It's not who's me. Yes, it makes me look who I am, but it doesn't make me any better or any less . . . He's sweet, my husband is a very sweet man, and I know there is not as many men out there. I really feel I've got the best . . . brought us closer, I know. But I did not know, you know, when a person tells you that they love you and they'll always stick by you, you never know until you test it on that. So, yes, I would say that it brought us closer because I know more than anything his love for me and his concern for me, it really takes a strong man to stand by his lady to go through this, because it is a lot. [Hanna]

Well, I'd say this. For me, I knew I had a good marriage, but, for me, it was also an affirmation, is that the right word, that my husband would stand by me no matter which way I decided. So it was good to know that he did that, because, like I said before, if he was so adamant about it, if he thought my breasts were that important, I would be very disappointed. So, I would say if your husband doesn't support you or, you know, tells you he's going to leave if you have this done, or whatever, I would say, you don't have a good relationship to start with. I mean, you could relate it to, say, a man had to testicular problems. If he had to have his testicles removed, would you leave him? [Kristen]

When It Was Good: What Mattered

A variety of actions by male partners were cited by women as having felt good through the decision making and the surgery. Some commented on how their spouse did not always know what to say or to do. This may well be a large problem for men in this circumstance, given the relative novelty of the surgery and its complex implications for the couple's physical and emotional relationship, but it is something that only the men could tell us and we do not have that data.

What did male partners do that was considered supportive to these women? They listened. This seemed very important, as women did not always have others with whom they could share their doubts, fears, or wishes and their partners were critical components, for many, in the decision of whether PM was right for them. In some cases, male partners participated actively in the decision making; in other cases, they made it clear that it was the woman's decision or they did not resist when the woman stated that she was the ultimate decision maker.

Partners did research about PM and went to doctor's visits with their wife or girlfriend. They held hands at crucial points; they complimented the woman on her good looks. They were good postsurgical caregivers—giving medication at the right time, taking care of the children, feeding the woman, caring for the house, etc. Some women openly refer to having gone through a "traumatic" event together as a couple, which had the potential to make them closer. In general, what was appreciated was joining the woman where she was in the process, whether it was in finding out what she needed to know, coming to a decision, or being there for her through the PM surgery. While it might sometimes be difficult to know exactly what a woman needed, the women in our study reported that they felt less alone with a partner who was not opposing them, but helping them. This need not mean that they avoided talking about what could be difficult about PM, but mostly just that they could talk about the issues with their male partner.

> So, and my husband was just fully supportive, in fact, as well and agreed. I think his term was, "It's a no-brainer to have this done." Oh, I did [talk it over with my husband]. We talked about it a lot, and he, I think, from day one thought, especially after my sister's diagnosis. I think before that we both were of the mind that, well, this is something I'll have to think about after we're done having our children . . . After my sister's diagnosis, he agreed completely that the sooner I could do it, the better . . . Yes, absolutely, absolutely. And continues to be [very supportive] . . . I would say the whole process of making the decision to have the surgery and then going through that, probably, if anything, may have brought us closer together because it really—we had to face our fears about this cancer in my family and what it potentially could do to our family and what we wanted to do about it. So, in that respect it brought us closer, I think.
>
> He's just, since the surgery, has continued to be really supportive of having it done, and, I think, makes a point of complimenting me on how I look and saying that he really likes it. Had he not been as supportive as he was, then I certainly would have talked to my doctors about what information can we give him to bring him on board, because I think it's important to have that support, if you have a spouse or someone close to you, to have the full support of that person, because I think you need that. I think I probably would have had it regardless [if he supported

me] because I was so convinced that it was the right thing. But it certainly made it much easier for me to make that decision and feel good about that decision by having his support. [Irene]

And even quiet partners could be seen as being valuable along a difficult journey. Ingrid describes her husband as "quiet, but loud." Afraid of losing her, but not strongly vocal about it, he was relieved postsurgery and they are "content" in their relationship.

He was supportive. Anything that I want to do was fine ... [How did your husband react?] Jeez, you know, I think it was uneventful ... My husband is a very—no, that's an oxymoron. He's quiet but he's loud. He doesn't say anything in front of me to upset me, and I think he's all right, except for "Oh, what you went through!" you know ... I think it's better [relationship with husband]. He was very much in the fear that, "Oh, God, I'm going to lose her." We're very content in our relationship, and the disfigurement that has happened, the scars, doesn't seem to bother him at all. [Ingrid]

The decision to undergo a prophylactic mastectomy involves painful examination of the risk that the woman could die at an early age of breast cancer. In some cases, this was openly discussed between the couple, while in other cases, it was more an unspoken background as the discussion focused on practical aspects of decision making. Some women concluded they would have made the same decision no matter what their partner had said. Others felt his support had been a necessary component of her willingness to undergo the surgery.

The entire time he was extremely supportive, always there. I don't think I could have gone through the whole—I'm not sure I would have done it, to tell you the truth, if I didn't have a good relationship with him, because I think I did it for us. [Laura]
     But when I went to my husband, he said, "I just want you here for the next fifty years." He said, "It doesn't matter to me ... He was very genuine, and he said, "You do what makes you feel most comfortable as you've always said." My husband just said, "I know that's going to make you feel the most relaxed in the end," and he goes, "that's all I want is you not to be sitting there worrying." No. I think my relationship is—well, I shouldn't say that. I guess I have a hell of a lot more respect of his love for me, I guess ... He really does love me beyond the physical. I always felt he did, but

I guess I think differently about him. I think, God, he's a great guy because he's been so great about this. I guess it puts him on another level in my mind, because he's really been there for me. [Julia]

My husband was the best. He went through everything with me. He came to see Dr. X with me and talked to her. You know, we had to go all the way to Boston from [distant state], and I had very young children at home, so it was really difficult. But he was with me throughout the whole thing, and he didn't want to decide this for me, which, he wanted it to be totally my decision with him being completely supportive of whatever that decision might be. So that's the way he was. He was great, and he still is.... The main thing is I'm still here, and I brought up my kids, and they're both in college, and I'm so thrilled that, and my husband is thrilled because if he didn't have me, he would have been the pits. He needed me. [Alice]

But even in the context of this positive emotional outcome, Julia harbors worries that her husband "misses the old me" and that this is a painful loss to him, which he avoids speaking about so as not to worry her.

I guess there's a part of me that he thinks something's lacking. Of course, he's never said that, but that's my insecurities. I don't think I'll ever, to my dying day, I'll feel like in his deep corners, he misses the old me. But, he really, and I do believe him, that he didn't want me fretting, he didn't want to risk my heart being taxed because I'd be questioning every mammogram.

Some couples seemed to have had more extensive talks and when they did, both the support and discussion of what was lost were discussed. This is significant since some of the narratives suggest that some women feel that they might not be able to hear about any sense of loss from their partners, that it might interfere with their feeling of being supported or make them feel guilty for taking away a source of pleasure from their partner. It is ultimately important that partners can acknowledge the individual losses and gains from this surgery, while focusing on the support for the decision they or she made.

I would say, I really would say that it hasn't changed. I'm sure, like he says, it's an adjustment, and that you have to kind of like refocus. But, you know, it hasn't. I don't think it's in any way made our relationship worse. Would he prefer that I had breasts? Yes, he'd prefer that I had breasts. But, it hasn't changed any. We still have very good sexual relationship and very strong love. It hasn't changed that. [Harriet]

Women spoke quite differently about the magnitude of impact of PM on their relationship with their partner. This may reflect differences in how deeply they discuss the physical and sexual changes as a result of the surgery. Some women expressed that the relationship was significantly changed while others that they felt it was unchanged, and several others noticed that there had been a temporary high or increased closeness, rather like that occurring after the birth of a baby, which subsided with time.

Just that I do think anybody considering this has to realize that it's going to have a tremendous impact [on your relationship]. I think a good relationship can withstand it, and one that has problems or a relationship where you're not used to working through difficulties of this sort, it's going to be challenging. There is no doubt about it. I think if you've got a great partner, they're probably going to be great about this. If there were problems, there are going to be problems. It's a big thing for us as a couple to go through. [Sandra]

In a supportive basis [my husband was involved]. He was behind me. My husband and nobody else was in the hospital with me ... My husband was very helpful ... Well, when I had my mastectomies, if anything, he probably was more supportive. Other than that, he is pretty much the same guy that he used to be. I don't think it has [changed my relationship]. I mean for better or for worse. [Sonia]

In the beginning, I think we were almost like closer because we'd had some time together and we'd gone through this traumatic thing. Now we're pretty much back to normal again. But it was like he was really nice to me after I had the kids, too, you know, but it wears off. [Meredith]

Other life experiences influence how the couple relates to the PM over time. The cancer experience of Rose's husband tempered his view of what she had chosen to do.

No, that it's different [the relationship]. That the relationship has changed. It's good to keep him involved, keeping him involved, made a big difference. He was very supportive. He wasn't crazy about it, but after he was diagnosed with testicular cancer, about four years ago, his feelings actually evolved about my surgery and now he is very understanding and he's very glad that I did it. [Rose]

When It Was Bad, It Was Very, Very Bad

Although the exception rather than the rule, some spouses failed the test of being supportive to their wives through the PM experience. In Valerie's case, she is clear that this decision came at a time when the relationship was already in deep trouble and her (now) ex-husband's reactions only contributed to her moving away from him.

My ex-husband really was not a help, unfortunately. At the time, we were having a lot of issues . . . But my battle was with my health, I thought, at the time. Even though my marriage was breaking up, that wasn't the focus for me. My ex even knew that. Then we came, actually, to an agreement that we just were not compatible. The divorce was not an adversarial divorce. We're actually good friends now; but we just weren't—It was inappropriate [his reaction to my decision]. All he was thinking of [was] what size implants I could have after surgery. So he's always been a jokester, and that was typical for him. But at the same time, it was very inappropriate. I was embarrassed. He actually said something like that in front of a surgeon and it kind of reinforced my sense of where my priorities actually were.

   Yes, he wasn't very supportive during the whole—the nine months—or almost a year, actually, until I made my decision. Then after the surgery, he was less supportive. I spent two weeks with my mother, right after the surgery, at her house and he pretty much took care of the kids at home. When I did go home, it was obvious that he really didn't take care of anything at the house . . . Not a single thing was done. . . . But, I mean, I was quite angry that he was so unsupportive to me in every arena. I mean, not just emotionally but physically. So now that I think of this, I'm thinking, "Why do I even talk to the man, after all this?" [Valerie]

While women were honest and open and reported a range of reactions to their PM surgery in their closest relationship, the message was that support from partners was highly valued and made a real difference to them. The sexual relationship might vary—and how much partners shared varied—but the emotional bonds were at least temporarily, and often permanently, strengthened for many couples.

The ultimate summary of a couple's sharing the satisfactions about the reduction in cancer fear following PM was offered by Sonia, "As a matter of fact, this year on February 25th, my husband and I celebrated the fact that I was alive instead of dead."

THE KIDS: IS MOM ALL RIGHT?

It is inevitable that children will continue to ask and wonder about the meaning of the PM surgery their mother has experienced for many years after the actual surgery. Daughters will especially also wonder about the implications of the family breast cancer history and their mother's decision about prevention in terms of the decision they may eventually face themselves. Children will also wonder how their mother has adjusted to her changed body and how she feels about the decision she made. This is normal considering that the mother's well-being is central to their own. How well children understand the preventive benefits and the family history of cancer will affect how much they worry. Even very young children know cancer is a serious disease that people can die from. If they have known individuals who have died from cancer, this will seem very real and possible to them, as we tend to overestimate the commonness of experiences we have had.[1] Even a discussion of cancer—if they do not fully understand—may raise or trigger their fear of cancer harming their mother. When the topic of cancer comes into a discussion with a child, remember to ask what they know and what have been thinking about their mother's surgery and her risk of cancer so that their fears can be appropriately addressed.

As children reach new developmental levels, learning about their mother's surgery is likely to affect them differently. A young school age child may be more concerned with the "differentness" of their mother's body, fears about the mother being away from home, or her being all right. When a daughter reaches adolescence and her own breasts begin to develop, her concern may focus on the emotional impact of such surgery on her mother and about whether her own breasts will remain healthy, or if she should have them eventually removed. An adolescent boy may be embarrassed about asking his mother about her breasts while at the same time interested in what it means to his mother to be without breasts. Letting children know that they can ask their questions and that they will receive an honest answer is the best way to overcome their natural hesitancy to bring up what they may fear is an upsetting topic.

Not really, not really. Maybe the first year after it was done, they did [her children ask questions]. "Are you all right? Is there anything we can do? Is everything okay? Are you okay?" Yes, that was their [my children's] major one concern, was I okay. [Janice]

While I was driving my son to the airport last summer, he was going to Florence for a semester abroad, and it was just me and him. He started asking me, "Mom, how do you feel about everything you went through in the last year?" I said, "I feel very lucky." He says, "How can you say that, because you don't have breasts?" I said, "I chose not to have breasts," I said, "But I think it gives me a better chance of living until I'm old." I said, "That's what's important to me. I want to see you kids grow old, and I want to see my grandchildren. And I feel real comfortable." He goes, "Well, what do you actually look like?" I said, "I actually, do you want to see?" He goes, "No." I said, "Okay, but I thought I'd ask you" . . . I had like a tank on, and I kind of like stretched, pushed my breasts down a little bit, and I said, "See those ribs? It's like that all the way down." He started laughing. He goes, "What about your nipples?" I said, "They took that, too." He goes, "Wow." He goes, "Really? Doesn't that bother you?" I said, "I think it bothers your father more than it bothers me." He goes, "Oh, don't go there, Mom." We started laughing. He said, "Okay, you answered all my questions. That's all I wanted to know." [Julia]

Jack [pseudonym] asked me if I could still get it [breast cancer]. He thinks about that. His brother doesn't ask me anything. I think it doesn't faze him at all. Jack asks me sometimes if that means that I'll never get it. He's very in tune with the fact that he never got to know his Grammy Emma [pseudonym], and he knew his Grammy Marie [pseudonym], which was my husband's mother, and he watched her die from cancer . . . I'm honest with him, you know. I tell him what the odds are, but, you know, that the likelihood is much less. He doesn't dwell on it, but every once in a while he'll ask me. Now they see that life has pretty much gone back to normal. He doesn't ask about it as much now as he did maybe the first year when I was still recovering from it. [Meredith]

Some of the women in the study noted that children can sometimes be sources of great comfort to their mothers as they come to understand the mother's action in a larger context.

One day my daughter and I put lipstick where they should have been [the nipples]. To them [my children], it was the most wonderful thing that I had an opportunity to check that ominous feeling of just waiting for it to happen . . . My son never [talks about the PM]. He forgets that it's even happened. He doesn't at all. My daughter, well, my daughter is twenty-seven. She's the baby. We just have a real good relationship. She started picking out low cut dresses for me, and you know, because that part doesn't show. You can wear a regular normal bathing suit. So, no, I don't. Bending over with a low cut or anything like that. As a matter of fact, people don't believe that you've had anything done, you know. She [my daughter] has made comments of "Is this what I've got to expect?" I told her I hope by the time she is of that age that the way things are moving it might not be as drastic a problem. [Ingrid]

Often when mothers have young children, they are unsure of how much to say to them about the PM surgery. The balance between being open and honest and frightening seems harder to find, as so much is unclear about what a young child understands about this complicated medical issue.

I just, basically, told them, "Mommy had surgery on the breast." They asked if it was cancer, and I told them no, because my oldest son says now, "Well, why did you do that?" I just tell him, "Because, I says, "you have to sit down and think of the statistics" . . . So he thanked me. He says, "Mommy, thank you for loving me." He says that I made a—he said it was a sacrifice that I made . . . I said, "Why do you say it's a sacrifice?" He says, "Well, Ma," he says, "you took something of yours away so that you could make sure that you're here with us." He says, "You've got a lot of love for us," and I thought that was nice. [Hanna]
  They were very young, they were three and five at the time. At some point I will want to tell them. It's important to tell them. . . . One of the problems about telling my daughters is that I really want them to enjoy their breasts, so I'm going to hold up on telling them until it's absolutely necessary. [Rose]

I told her [my daughter] when she saw the scars. She said, "What happened?" I mean she was little, four or something. I told her that, and she's always known about her aunt dying and that she had something that grew inside her, that was cancerous, and that grew inside her and that made her really sick. And that there was a chance that that could happen to me, but I didn't want that to happen to me, so I asked the doctors to remove the insides of my breasts so that they couldn't get sick the way hers did. So, now I'm safe, and what's left over are these scars, but that I'm okay and that nothing would happen to me because of that. She asked if it hurt. I said no.

We've, of course, talked about it many times since then. Actually, she has asked if she's going to have to do this. Well, I've said that every year everything changes, with medicine, and I didn't think she would have to worry. I really don't want her to worry, so I tell her, "No, I had to do this because it was my sister. It's your aunt, and that's not the same kind of relationship. So, you don't have to worry about this. And medicine changes all the time, and someday there may be no cancer at all for anybody. So people who have all different kinds of diseases won't have to deal with this, we hope, by the time you get older." That's extremely optimistic, but I certainly don't want her carrying anything around right now. [Sandra]

When daughters become young adults, the issues of their own cancer prevention come up even more forcefully which is often difficult for both mother and daughter. When a daughter is pregnant, a mother sometimes avoid the discussion of their own surgery or of the implications of the daughter's risks so as not to interfere with the happy anticipation of the new baby.

I actually didn't tell my daughter about my decision and what I was going to have. I think I waited until after she had the baby. I don't think I said anything to her until then. I told my son a little bit earlier, as long as he promised not to tell anybody . . . Yes. My daughter asked me how I'm feeling, and my son has pretty much forgotten it. My daughter wants, actually, she's pregnant right now with her third. She wants to have her family. She doesn't want it to be part of what she has to think about right now, but I would be willing to bet that within about five years she'll make some decisions. [Laura]

A mother may also have a message she strongly wants to convey to her daughters related to their own health and how to protect it. As genetic testing becomes more common, there will be more families where mothers are aware of their daughter's actual or potential high risk for breast cancer. The mother may want to underscore the daughter's need to be proactive, as she has been. It may be difficult to know how children of different ages hear this message; some may accept it and others may want not to hear about it until they are older. Some daughters may simply feel that prophylactic surgery is not an acceptable option for them and this can cause disagreements or even rifts in some families.

> I informed my daughters on it and told them to be very aggressive on theirs [their breasts] . . . I talked with them prior to that, when my mother was dying . . . I talked to them that I was going to have this because I didn't want to get cancer, because I've had enough. They just accepted it. They have been well versed on all of that, with their grandmother and everything . . . I just told them that the biggest thing is for them to be aggressive themselves, because high risk tumors are in the family. Just to keep a heads up on all of that. Yes, they watch themselves, yes. They are very pro into watching themselves. They're really not a candidate for mammograms yet, but they do breast checks themselves. [Vicky]
>
> I just want her to be comfortable with her body, with bodies, period. That's also why I've never, you know, I don't parade naked, but if I'm in the bathroom and she comes in and that's how she saw me the first time. I mean she walks into the bathroom and there I am changing or getting dressed or whatever. That's when she would see that I've got the scars. I didn't want her to be afraid, and I didn't want her to be afraid to ask. I didn't want her to keep her questions to herself. I would urge that on any parent, to just be sort of—you don't want to give too much information, things that aren't appropriate for their age. You always have to remember what their age is. Don't fool yourself into thinking, "Oh, they're just kids. They don't think or notice." Because they do, I mean I'm positive they do. I'm living testament to that. [Sandra]

SISTERS

It is with sisters that much of the family drama about hereditary cancer is played out. Studies have shown that both the most positive and some of the most negative interactions about hereditary cancer takes place between sisters.[2, 3] Perhaps, the most typical pattern currently is that a mother develops breast cancer, is genetically tested and finds she has a *BRCA1/2* mutation, and then tells her daughters (if they are teenagers or older) and often other female relatives as well, with the hope they will consider testing to find out if they are mutation carriers. The discussion happens soon after disclosure.[4] Sisters, if they are close, are likely to share their reactions, their plans, and their fears. They may talk together and share information from their doctors about what they can do to protect themselves against breast cancer. They may go to doctor's visits together and may support each other in the decisions they make about whether to have PM surgery or not. Sometimes, spouses feel left out as their wives look more to their sister or sisters for support about hereditary cancer and the decisions they have to make. However, the closeness between sisters does not always translate into similar action steps when the specter of hereditary cancer is raised. Some sisters who consider themselves to be close may decide this is an area where they do not wish to be confidants. Usually, the only guarantee is that there will be intensity in the interactions between sisters!

When breast cancer is diagnosed in a woman, it can be very frightening for the woman's sisters. Unlike when a mother has breast cancer, the age difference does not act as an emotional buffer. It is certainly frightening to have a mother develop breast cancer, but a woman can always rationalize, "Well, that may happen to me too, when I get to that age." When the woman with cancer is someone whose genes are very closely aligned to yours (even closer than a parent) and they are approximately the same age, the reality is, if they can develop cancer, you can too, which is much more frightening. Thus, much of the intensity between sisters has to do with this fear. One sister may lecture another about what she should do based on fear. Another, out of fear, may not want to hear what a doctor told her sister. Or, in the best of circumstances, sisters may be able to help each other conquer the fear by being there for each other through learning about their breast cancer risks and making and carrying out their individual decisions with regard to their risks. When there are differences of opinion and difficulty even talking about the implications of hereditary cancer risk, it is often perceived that the other is not hearing or thinking that this is an important topic, when, in fact, fear most often is responsible for disrupting communication between sisters.

> Well, the only one I would discuss it with would be my sister, and she has somewhat of a denial attitude, and her breasts are very important to her. They're important to her husband. She would never have that done. She's just in kind of denial and just wants to take her chances, which to me is a little foolish, but she does get herself regular checks . . . There was times when she couldn't be there for me because she was so scared. [Kristen]
>
> I mentioned it [genetic testing], and they [my sisters] said, "Oh, hogwash," basically. They don't want to know just—they just don't think it's a possibility, I think. Because one sister did have a mass that was benign. The other sister just won't even bother going for mammograms. She totally has her head in the sand about this. I guess sometimes I get frustrated and other times I just have to re-sign myself to the fact that they are adults, and they're going to have to make their own decisions about things like that. [Valerie]

In a family where the sisters are supportive and agree on what they think is right for them to do regarding their breast cancer risk, there can be a great deal of information sharing as well as social support. For Beth, who had four sisters, PM surgery seemed to be an expectation and even her sister who "did not have the marker" had a prophylactic mastectomy.

> So the one sister with the markers went in. She had hers done, I don't know, maybe three, four years ago. Well, she had a son and nursed him, so she must have done it four years ago. Then my older sister who did not have the marker was still scared about it. She went in and did it anyway . . . Yes, but she's, the one sister that's left, is much younger than we are. So, let's see. The three older ones were all two years apart. I went first, and my older sister went, and then my, then the third oldest went. Then Annabelle [not real name] is still, she's thirty-three, and she's actually, she just had her first baby, so I think she's waiting a little bit. [Beth]

Having sisters (or other close relatives) who have undergone prophylactic mastectomies means that a woman participates in a sort of a dress rehearsal for what happens with surgery and what some of the outcomes of reconstructive choice are in real life. Many women without such support know no one who has undergone a PM and it can be much more frightening and lonely as they make their choices. A sister in the former example would be likely to hear what went well and what did not, how long recovery was and what it was like. This familial relationship can then be helpful in ways that a relationship with a medical professional may not be able to be. Of course, on the other hand, these professionals are familiar with the entire range of PM experiences and, therefore, may know the range of likely outcomes, not just the one or two idiosyncratic ones which occur for the sisters in a particular family.

Any individual case must be taken as just that—one possible outcome. Yet, just the opportunity to observe how that case turns out may influence a woman's choice about whether this is or is not a path she wants to take. In either case, it is probably useful for a woman to do some thinking about how she is or is not like the woman who has undergone PM and to ask herself—and perhaps her surgeon or plastic surgeon—if any of the ways in which she is different are likely to affect the outcome of the surgery. However, being able to watch the post-surgical progress of a close relative is an empowering experience, making very clear that it all resolves in the end, even if sometimes the cosmetic result is not exactly what had been anticipated, or the time frame a little different from what had been expected.

> I have two other sisters who were very supportive. In fact, I have another sister who has had it done . . . Yes. They don't live here, they live in other states. But they, too, have been involved in going to breast care specialists and things. My one sister, same kind of thing, started to have issues. She does not have children yet. She made this decision. My other sister, who is a little bit younger, same thing, has two children, and is just starting to talk about it now. I have shown her my scars and whatever her feelings are and whatever, she's really thinking seriously about it . . . I think they, having watched me going through it and how I feel afterwards, that it wasn't anything detrimental. I look fabulous, so there's no ugly scarring or anything like that. Just that I feel so good about it, which was just the surprising thing, too. [Kate]

Some cancer centers will link a woman considering PM to another woman who has undergone the procedure. This relationship can also be empowering and encouraging, but the woman contemplating the surgery must also ask questions of the woman who has had PM to determine how they are alike and different and to remember that one experience is not always the same as another. While this may seem contradictory, the real life knowledge of a woman who has gone through the surgery and come out the other side is in itself very reaffirming and comforting. Seeing the outcomes may help a woman decide not only if she wants PM surgery, but also what type of reconstruction will fit her needs and her lifestyle and personality.

Probably my sister who was [the most influential person]—well, both my sisters, the one who diagnosed and my youngest sister who is actually an OB/GYN. And then my husband. My sister who was diagnosed with the cancer said, "You know, it's time. We know what we're up against now." She said to both myself and my youngest sister, "You guys should have the surgery." Again, I think I was influenced by my sister who had the cancer diagnosis and had the bilateral mastectomy, and she did not initially have any reconstruction because she was going through radiation and didn't want the reconstruction, particularly the implants, to interfere with that in any way. So, talking with her, I realized she felt, she said, she really wished she did have something there. That she did feel kind of funny and like a boy walking around. It was just kind of strange. So, she really said, you know, and I think she intended at some point to go back in and have the reconstruction done if that could be done.

So, talking with her, I said, "You know, I'm young. I have a lot of years in front of me, hopefully," and I wanted to consider reconstruction for that reason. Then, I actually did reconstruction with implants as opposed to the flap, because my youngest sister made the decision and had the kind of the natural reconstruction done and had some complications. [She's] Very, very pleased with the results, but it was kind of an ordeal for her. She spent a lot of time in the hospital and is actually going to have to go back in to have some dead tissue removed at some point. I think I thought, for me, that the implants would be fine and it's much easier and it's worked out really well. It's wonderful. [Irene]

When there are major differences in views and where the communication is not supportive, it can be very difficult between sisters. Especially in families where other women have suffered from and/or died from breast cancer, these are emotionally-loaded topics. PM requires such a global assessment of what stage the woman is in her life and what the risks are and how to live with them, that it is understandable why even sisters would come to very different conclusions. But often, sisters feel it should not be that way, that they should all see the risks and benefits of PM in the same manner. The motivation is often very well meaning, but the conclusions may be both different and difficult to hear. Fear again is a major factor. A woman who is convinced that PM is the right decision for her also wants her sister to have her risks reduced as much as her own. She wants her sister to be spared the anguish of breast cancer. Thus, it may feel wrong to her that her sister seems unwilling to consider PM, that the views the sister has about the integrity of her body, her willingness to live with mammograms and MRIs rather than surgery, seem heretical to the woman who is opting for PM, perhaps at a different point in her life than her sister. Patience and tolerance for these differences may be short-circuited by the fear of breast cancer. The insistence on PM as the only way to defeat this disease may be perceived as arrogance and as a continuation of an unwanted older sister role.

I have a sister that I've talked with about it. She said she would do it if her doctor says for her to do it. Right now, they've got her, the doctor that she's seeing over at [hospital name] thinks that I shouldn't have done it. Really, I have a hard time to want to get into topics with people on it, unless they are going through it, because people—I don't know. It's hard when you have a family member say, "Why did you do such a thing?" They just don't quite understand where I'm at or where I was at or where I'm at today. [Hanna]

And I have to say I did not get support from my sisters at all. At all, which was hurtful. I think it's because they're afraid. They just don't want to go there with me. They said, "Well, I think you're a little overzealous." [Julia]

They're all wishing that they'd listened to me, followed me when I'd had that same cyst [unclear] but they opted on something else . . . Then what I had, they all wished that they had followed me, but I said, "You have to make your decisions what you're ready to take on." [Janice]

Silence is the response in some families where fear does not allow for differences of opinion among siblings about PM surgery. Their shared experience leads them to very different conclusions and the differences do not allow them to tolerate the views of the other as reasonable. This can be a very painful process.

I didn't speak to my sister about it. I just went ahead and did it . . .
My own sister has never even been for a mammogram. She can't

talk about it. My family has had a very, very diverse reaction to my surgery. No, no, I have never spoken to my sister about my experience. She's never asked me. We went to my cousin's funeral in May. My cousin was buried because of breast cancer. The gene result had not come in. My sister, as that time, knew that I'd had a prophylactic mastectomy, and she completely avoided the whole subject. She can't talk to me about it. Yet, she's at the same level of risk as I was, and she sat on my mother's bed and was told that she should have a prophylactic mastectomy. So she has had the identical experience I have had, other than where my experience parted from hers coming to Boston.

But the fact that at the time I was seeing [doctor's name] in Boston, I went to my sister, and I had to speak to her about the cousin on my father's side of the family that [the doctor] wanted to have tested. At that time, she said, "Why are you doing this?" I said, "Because I'm looking into the possibility of a prophylactic mastectomy," and she just completely flipped out and the conversation ended right there. In light of that conversation, she told me that she had never had a mammogram, and she was forty-five when that conversation occurred. [Joyce]

Sometimes seeing the result of PM surgery can help resolve the tensions with family members. Beth's sisters did try to support her, despite prior differences of opinion, but the real resolution came after the surgery when they saw how pleased she was with her results.

Yes, you know, it's only because I think we all [sisters] sort of hung out. They came up to visit me the day before I went in, or a couple of days before. We all went downtown and had a, you know, whatever, chit-chat and lunch, a great girls' day. Then I think once I did it and we saw, you know, the other end of it, it was all fine. Everybody was a little more relaxed about it, including my father. He just seemed to be much more at ease with the whole thing. [Beth]

OTHER RELATIVES

Once the PM surgery is accomplished, questions still remain about who will be told, who will be supportive or not, and what might the impact of the surgery be on family relationships. Parents, sisters,

brother, cousins, aunts, sisters-in-law, prospective daughters-in-law—
many women are surprised by the range of family members whom
they may feel they want to tell or should tell about their own experience. On the other hand, the desire for privacy may push a woman in
the other direction, away from telling everyone she thinks might have
a medical interest in her condition, at least initially.

> What do you mean by family? I told my parents. I told my imme-
> diate family. I told my siblings and my parents and my husband.
> My children, obviously, did not know. They were too little. But,
> like, I have sister-in-laws and things that I'm close with. I'm very
> close to my husband's brother's wife that doesn't know. I have
> close friends that do not know. I just chose not to tell a lot of peo-
> ple because I felt like once you tell—I didn't want everyone to
> know. I didn't want everyone to know. I've got a daughter. I just
> didn't want it to be out there, that it would be public. So, I just
> basically told my immediate family. [Harriet]

Joyce felt if she told many people in her family and some disagreed
with her decision, it might make it harder for her to move ahead
with the surgery. Once she had the surgery, she chose an aunt, whom
she felt carried authority in this area with other family members
and asked her to inform their relatives about the surgery she had
undergone.

> Reactions to my decision to have a prophylactic mastectomy? I
> actually only told two people that I had made the decision. I told
> my brother, and he was very supportive. I very purposefully did
> not speak to any other members of my family, because I didn't
> want anybody to shake my resolve.

Women in our study spoke about how the passage of time had
changed who they told and how they felt about sharing the information and with whom they felt comfortable sharing it. And the passage
of time also changed the responses they received from their relatives.
As their female relatives, especially the younger ones, came into life
stages where PM was more likely—once they were married, had their
children, and were approaching ages at which breast cancer had
appeared in their families—they seemed both more interested and
more eager to learn about PM.

They [my cousins] thought we were sort of—they just weren't crazy about the idea. They didn't want to know. But I think now that they've had kids and both of them are married, they're changing their mindsets, so they're all starting to go through the procedures. [Beth]

Time may be needed for some women to recognize both the extent of the risks and reduction in that risk which PM surgery offers. Even with such recognition, some women may not want to consider PM for a variety of reasons. This is important to remember if relatives react with resistance or even hostility, especially if they are individuals to whom the risk of breast cancer and knowledge of the benefits of PM may be new information.

I think, certainly, I had some family members, even on my husband's side of the family, who, initially, thought, "Is she nuts? She's going to go get her breasts cut off." But, I think once I talked to them and they understood the full extent of the situation, I mean they were aware of my family history, and then once they became aware of the genetic situation, I think everyone once they understood the full situation and what the real risks were, everyone realized that this was a good thing. It makes a lot of sense. [Irene]

Fathers and Brothers

Male relatives—fathers and brothers—are least frequently told about genetic test results[4] and probably also about PM. Women are more comfortable talking with female relatives whom they usually assume understand more about the feelings brought about by the decision to have surgery and the subsequent lack of natural breasts. We have little information about what males, including husbands, feel about PM and especially about their feelings during the decision making. Most of what we do know comes from the reports from women. However, it is not always true that male relatives have little impact or are avoided in discussions about prophylactic surgery. Male relatives who are physicians are often asked for advice and some others manage to convey their willingness to be consulted and to have their opinions heard.

Well, my brother's a doctor in Boston, and my family had some-how—he had been contacted by another doctor who was a distant relative. He, my brother, like started gathering information, and that was the beginning how we found out . . . My brother had a lot of influence as a doctor. We discussed it quite a bit. [Hanna]

Fathers may find the prospect of a daughter undergoing PM quite difficult and for many father-daughter pairs, this is a difficult subject to discuss. Alice looked back, however, grateful for her father's honesty in sharing his true feelings about her plans for the surgery.

Brothers, too, may feel fear for the sister considering PM and may come to the conclusion that the surgery is barbaric and should be opposed.

It's funny, because my family—well, my brother John was pretty supportive. But my brother Tommy was actually angry about me doing it. He thought I was mutilating myself and it was unnecessary or it wouldn't work anyway. Then like a month before I was hooked up for surgery, stuff came out about Tamoxifen . . . So my brothers were calling me, going, "You don't have to do this. They have Tamoxifen now." I'm like, "It's not that simple, you know." It was funny. My husband was very supportive, and one of my brothers was pretty supportive. But my father and my older brother were actually sort of angry at me for doing it. It was kind of weird, and it wasn't really until about a year after I had the surgery that they came out, finally, with some research on it and showed that it [PM] actually does seem to be helpful. Now they'll say, probably, that I did the right thing, but at the time, they were, I don't know, kind of adamantly calling me and telling me not to do it. . . . I never really quite understood. I think he just was horrified. [Meredith]

WHAT ARE FRIENDS FOR?

Individuals inside one's family are more likely to know about PM because there are multiple reasons for telling them. Not only does telling them let them know about important things happening to a family member, but there also are often "modeling" reasons—wanting to model for them that risk-reducing surgery is a reasonable alternative to reliance on screening for those women who are at high risk for breast cancer and who are comfortable considering PM surgery. Relatives, even those with whom a woman may not have been all that close before information about hereditary cancer risk came to light, may already have shared information about the risk, about genetic testing, or information about doctors or genetic counselors, so it may be an extension of those conversations which leads to discussion about PM. Also, within families the telephone method of communication where one relative tells another who then tells another is fairly common. While not always acceptable or comfortable, it is not unusual for relatives to know a good deal about each other by this method, even if they are not particularly close.

Support from Friends

With friends, the reasons for telling or not telling of the decision to have PM may well be different and the acceptability of knowing personal information through others may be less acceptable. Especially (but not only) in families where there is little support available from relatives, women often rely on one or more close friends to help them manage both the practical and the emotional crises which surgery occasions. Close friends can be a tremendous support for a woman before and after her surgery.

I remember everybody coming and bringing in suppers and leaving me stuff. I had a lot of support. I had a lot of support, you know, taking the kids to school, whatever. [Janice]
My girlfriend came down from Canada to take care of me . . . She's like a sibling. I had wonderful, wonderful care at home after the surgery. [Joyce]

Privacy

While telling others about PM can initiate much-wanted support, it can also open a woman to unwanted observation or scrutiny. Many women want to share their plans with close friends, and co-workers, there may also individuals whom a woman does not want to knows about her prophylactic mastectomy. A woman may hold off on telling some friends for fear of whom they, in turn, might tell in a widening circle which includes people she wouldn't want to know. Women may also want to avoid difficult experiences their children might confront if schoolmates learn about the surgery from their parents; even if she is friendly with the parents of other children, she may opt not to talk about the surgery with them. Women also say they do not want

to be stared at and they do not want people they hardly know talking
their breast surgery.

> I really needed to keep my privacy at work and so I didn't really
> want people looking at me or thinking that I looked different,
> so in that regard it was very different for me. [Rose]

How the women in our study define the private sector from the
public sector in their lives varied considerably. For some women,
the people they work with were definitely on the outside of the line
marked "Private." Other women gathered a great deal of support from
their openness with work colleagues.

> Let me put it to you this way. I'm a very private person. What
> goes on with my life is nobody else's business. Other than that,
> my immediate family, being my brother and sister, and close
> friends, they knew all about it. People that I worked with or any-
> thing like that, it's none of their business. [Sonia]

In contrast, Ingrid felt:

> No, everyone at work was completely supportive.... everybody
> at work and everything was just great. [Ingrid]

Lack of Support

Occasionally, a woman in the study reported a strong lack of support from friends about her decision to undergo a PM. In such a case,
a woman had to consider how much to invest in bringing her friends
along until they could at least understand her reasons for going forward with the surgery. Some women felt that friends who are not
themselves at risk for hereditary breast cancer cannot really know the
stress a high risk woman feels. Julia mentioned that "I felt terrible
opposition from my friends and my peers."

Other women take a more open view, thinking that there is no reason to keep silent about this surgical procedure any more than about
any other medical procedure.

> But my friends knew, people at work knew, and my relatives.
> They were just kind of matter of fact about it. I mean, nobody
> was devastated, "Oh, my God," you know. [Valerie]

I definitely felt support. I think everyone in my immediate family, and close friends, everyone knew I was going to have the surgery. [Irene]

I'm not Brave

For some women, the support they received from friends went beyond what they felt they deserved. They and their friends saw the rationale and motivation from a different perspective; they did not feel that they had been "brave," as their friends saw them.

I just have to say it was one of the easiest decisions I've ever made. And how many times people said to me, "Oh, you're so brave," I thought, "You're crazy." This is not the brave decision of somebody who It's not even a decision. I just thought if I can do this, I'm going to do this. It was so easy. [Sandra]

The reaction of Kate's best friend was,

"I cannot believe how brave you are, and that you just went through this." I said, "But you don't understand how good I feel now, how I felt like I had to do that." It wasn't bravery. It was sure self-preservation as far as I was concerned. [Kate]

I tell people that I hate when people look at me and say, "Oh, you're so brave." I'm not; I just did what I felt I had to do. Because I don't think of it as a brave thing . . . I could understand other people—regular people's point of view on the thing. But when you're facing the choice of, "Am I playing Russian roulette and I could die any minute from having a bad tumor, or get rid of these breasts?" [Fay]

The thing that I thought was weird was that everybody thought I was so brave. That was a weird thing to me because I thought I'm a coward to do this. Do you know what I mean? I'm doing it because I'm scared shitless. I looked at all these women like my patient advocate, the women in the hospital who actually had cancer and were struggling with that, and what my mom had gone through, and those women are brave. They have to be. But with me, it was like I'm chicken, and I want to get this done before I get it. . . . I remember when I went in to get the surgery that day in the operating room there were people waiting for me because they'd read my chart the day before and they were all there telling me about someone they knew who'd done it or how brave they thought I was being, and I thought, "That's really weird, because I'm here because I'm really scared." Like I was more scared not to do it than I was to do it. [Meredith]

The fact that prophylactic mastectomy remains relatively rare made some women feel that they would be looked at as different or "freakish" in ways they did not want to experience, so this became another reason for not telling friends. Sandra seemed worried that it was demanding too much of acquaintances or work mates to help her through the death of her sister and then ask them to support her through surgery. It was as if she was afraid she would be pitied and she did not want that to happen.

I've gone to therapy, sort of about the feeling of there's the loss of my sister and everything's been affected, like being hexed almost. Like why did this happen to her and to our whole family? You start to feel like there's a freakish quality, too. When your grief is so big and so outside what your normal experience was before, I just didn't want to have to explain to people. So, I shared it with a friend and a few people, but they were all sort of close circle ... So, I have to say, I did get a lot of positive reinforcement. "You're doing the right thing." Some of those people that went, "Oh, you're so brave, and when I said I didn't feel brave, but it was nice to get support in any form.

Telling Easier Afterwards

There was, for some women in the study, a change after the surgery which made them feel that it was much easier then to be open to telling people about the surgery. In some cases, this reversed their previous feelings and represented considerable movement in their comfort zone defining the line between private and public.

It's interesting, but there's a big difference when you tell people after the fact than before the fact. [Rose]
   You know what; I'm a pretty private person. I didn't tell any of my friends beforehand to get any kind of feedback. Also, because, if you've gone through a death in your family, you know that people look at you in a different way, you can feel that. Unless you know of somebody who has gone through a similar thing with you, it's a tremendous thing to lay on somebody else, I have

found in my life, having lost two parents and a sister. It's a big thing to lay on somebody who maybe hasn't gone through that in their life. They can't possibly understand. So I am more comfortable not discussing those things. Unless someone else has gone through that, then I know they can relate to that kind of thing. So I'm pretty private that way. But the funny thing is, after I had it done, I couldn't wait to tell them. My friends, yes. I didn't tell anybody at work or anything, but my very, very close friends, I told them. I said, "I feel so terrific." It wasn't an issue afterwards. Before, yes. It was a very private kind of thing. [Kate]

Like so much about PM, deciding *who* to tell *what* to *when* is a very private matter. For some women, it is a matter of wanting to seem as normal as possible, and not to evoke pity or a sense of difference. Conversely, others find it normal to share events of this magnitude with others and they welcome the practical and emotional gains which social support can bring.

CHAPTER 8

What It Cost: Physical and Emotional Consequences of Surgery

Women undergoing bilateral prophylactic mastectomy (PM) without a diagnosis of cancer are not ill. They seem to expect that surgery will go easily and predictably, and that after a brief recovery period, they will feel good physically as they adjust emotionally to their changed body. As mentioned in Chapter 5, as women approach the day of surgery, they do not seem focused on worry about postoperative pain. After surgery, pain seems to come as an unwelcome surprise in many cases after the months of doctor visits, decision making, and informing family and friends which culminated in the decision for surgery.

The reports of women's postoperative pain, complications, and disappointments were in marked contrast to what they would say about their overall satisfaction with their decision and with the surgery. The physical experience was described as having felt quite real and unpleasant, at least for a while, and yet, the freedom from the "sword of Damocles," the fear of breast cancer which has hung over them, predominated. For those women who had feared that they had already waited too long before having surgery, the knowledge that the removed breast tissue was free of cancer was a great relief. Other women focused on their postsurgery freedom from the many screening visits, which had often been accompanied by high anxiety about whether this would be the time the cancer would be found. In general, women felt they were moving away from the medicalization of their livesand this was highly prized. Breast cancer worries were moved to the "back burner" in their lives, but the price women paid willingly for this freedom was considerable. The stories of their experience with PM necessarily includes telling about what they were surprised by adversely, what they struggled with during the postsurgery period, and how it affected their overall thinking about their decision.

The women in our study had experienced a number of different surgical and reconstructive procedures. Most of these women either had implants (silicone or saline), TRAM (Transverse Rectus Abdominus Musculocutaneous) flap surgery, or no reconstruction. Our focus here is on the women's retrospective emotional experience of surgery, not on the specifics of what side effects were experienced with a certain types of reconstruction. That information is very important to the decision making process to those now seeking a prophylactic mastectomy, but it is better provided by physicians or surgeons who have deeper and broader knowledge and experience in the range of surgical outcomes and their management. In addition, some of these women had their surgeries some years ago and the options offered now (or in the future) may be quite different than what these women experienced. We are not in a position to say if these are typical or broadly atypical side effects and sequelae of surgery. What we present is what the women told us they felt and how they dealt with the pain and other effects of the PM. We think this information provides context to their stories and also gives other women now considering PM some idea of what to ask of oncologists, surgeons, and plastic surgeons.

PAIN

Several women described the immediate, postPM discomfort as being "like having a semi [truck] on top of your chest." Although obviously unpleasant, this feeling was relatively short-lived, but as the surgical anesthetic wore off, the pain was quite real.

Coming out of it [the surgery], I think I was in more pain than I expected to be, and that might have been that I just probably wasn't focusing on that aspect of it, because I know the doctors had explained to me that, "Yes, it's going to hurt. You're going to be on some pain medication and some restrictions in terms of your movements." And I think I was just so focused on getting it done that I wasn't really focused on what it was going to be like after I had it done. I was definitely in a fair amount of pain and just very, very tired. I know that's common after a major surgery, so I think I was kind of surprised. I'm a very active person, and, of course, having two little kids in the house and everything, you're on the go all the time. So, I was surprised at the amount of time I felt like I needed to be just laying on the couch . . . But I needed to do that and rest. I think I'd have to say I felt pretty much the same throughout. I was sure of my decision going in and even after I had it done, I think I was kind of stunned by the amount of pain involved. But, when you're cutting off a part of your body, I guess that's to be expected. So, I think I still, afterwards, I still felt good about the decision and had no regrets. [Irene]

[How was it for you right after surgery?] Horrible. I had no clue how bad I would feel. Very. I had reactions to the pain and couldn't stop vomiting. For the entire days I was there, it was terrible. The pain was horrible. It was much, much worse than I would have ever guessed. [Laura]

Oh, yes, I did [have pain], but, you know, the usual. When somebody cuts you up, you're going to hurt. But, no, it was worth it to me. [Kristen]

Other kinds of postsurgical discomfort included having bad reactions to the anesthesia or nausea from the morphine received for pain. Some women mentioned the difficulty they had immediately postsurgery with standing.

Nobody prepared me for the fact that I wasn't going to be able to stand up straight or that I was going to be short of breath for two weeks because I wouldn't have any blood. That stuff scared me. [Meredith]

Meredith reasoned that perhaps the doctors were afraid to tell her clearly about the postsurgical pain because they might have thought she would avoid surgery if she knew it would be painful.

As with any surgery, there can be hospital experiences which do not meet with expectations. Valerie described a too hasty withdrawal by the doctors of the morphine which was treating her postoperative pain, which led her to have very high anxiety. She did feel the nurses then took good care of her, closing the shades, turning off the lights, eliminating as much noise as possible. "It probably took about an hour for me to get to feel that it wasn't a heart attack and I wasn't going to die."

A few women in our study spoke of continuing pain after the surgery.

> I have pain all the time. There isn't a time when I don't, and it's the kind of thing where if I eat very much, if I'm even slightly bloated, it feels so bad that at times I almost feel like doubling up. Yet, I function, I work all day at work, but there are times, too, when I sit in the chair and wonder if I'm going to be able to stay in that position long enough to get through my therapy session. [Laura]

Yet, others were struck by how little pain they had or how quickly it resolved.

> Actually, I think it was a little bit easier. I didn't have as much pain as I kind of expected I would. [Emily]

> Also, this is real important. People think, "Ooh, they cut off your breasts. That must hurt. That must hurt." You picture somebody losing something like a leg or an arm, there's a sense of a pain, physical pain that you imagine. It's really not. As I tell people, I think in some ways when I had my wisdom teeth out, that hurt more, and I always use that image. That really was—that just hurt so bad. [Fay]

> I'm a healthy fit person. I found that the surgery was not hard at all. It was the biggest procedure I had ever had, but it only was a two- to three-day stay in the hospital. What I was not prepared for was how painful it was and the discomfort I felt immediately after. In fact, one week later I was already riding the T [the Boston subway], so that's how fast I recovered, but that next day, I just wasn't prepared for the pain that I felt. [Rose]

COMPLICATIONS

The rates of postsurgical complication and what is referred to as "unanticipated re-operation" in prophylactic mastectomy and subsequent reconstruction is high. Many women seem not to have anticipated this and were frustrated by the ways in which complications extended the period of time over which they had to deal with the physical consequences of PM. Medical complications which were reported by women in our cohort included: engorgement because the surgical drains became blocked, frozen shoulder requiring physical therapy, and limited range of motion in both arms.

> I would say it was probably—I mean it was several months certainly before I felt like I had really kind of full range of motion. I know in terms of my strength and lifting and particularly lifting above my head, it took—I mean I know it was in the range of months, maybe even six months, before I really felt like I had full strength. I know today even there are some things like opening cans, like for whatever reason, that torque, I feel not as strong as I used to be, and maybe that's just age and nothing to do with this. [Irene]

Other medical complications included rheumatoid problems related to silicone implants, necrosis (dying) of some tissue necessitating removing expanders, staph infection, the need for a blood transfusion, bladder leak following surgery (woman relates it to here catheter); shooting arm pain, swollen fingers (attributed by the woman to post-surgery virus); numbness.

> Well, there was still a lot of numbness. But if you touched, I couldn't feel—I couldn't feel my hand and my breast, if I touched it. But probably just underneath the skin it was like electrical current, probably shooting but in every direction... It was the most annoying thing I think I ever experienced. It wasn't pain. Well, I expected numbness but not that electrical activity. I swear to God, there was like a car battery attached to my chest, and the current was just constantly running through... Yes, yes. I remember calling the plastic surgeon and telling him about it; and he said, "You need to get a face cloth and rub the tissue vigorously." The thought of anything touching the tissue made my skin crawl. I couldn't put clothes over it. The thought of having to rub vigorously even didn't sit well with me. But I bit the bullet and I did it, and it took probably a month before that sensation went away. I thought it would never, ever go away. [Valerie]

Other sequelae of surgery, which do not qualify as "complications" included the following symptoms as described by Fay.

> I also found that the cold air as you stepped outdoors, that now not having that extra meat on my chest, the cold air would make the pectoral muscles contract and flutter. It was a funny, sort of painful feeling and I actually still get that feeling now. Now it

doesn't hurt; it feels weird. I step outdoors and it's cold. It's like your pecs are right there and they will just suddenly contract, and it's a funny little fluttery, weird tightness.

Some women had no physical complaints postsurgery and nothing hampering their activity after surgery. Janice reported that "I was one of the lucky ones that had no problems, no swelling, no armpit swelling, or arms swelling, or anything like that."

UNANTICIPATED REOPERATION

While some surgeries are planned as part of the reconstruction of the breasts, if problems develop, they may necessitate additional, usually minor, surgeries. Depending on the woman's expectations and mindset, these additional surgeries may be very frustrating or simply seen as part of the recovery process.

Well, I guess it's not major [problems with the reconstruction], but I had to have five operations, and there are several operations when you have the expander put in, you know, this saline thing, and the implants. You know, you have to do it in steps, but I had a problem because one of my temporary implants got infected. So I had to have the operation to put them, then the operation to take one out, and then to wait a while and to have the operation to put the temporary back in again, and then when they come out, put the permanent, and then do the nipple. So that was five. [Laughs] Yes, it was real drag, you know, the [reconstruction] infection part, because it was scary. It was not knowing what's going to happen. My doctor tried to reassure me. "You know, even though this has happened, it's just going to take longer, and you'll be fine," which I was . . . So it was half a year or something. [Alice]

Shortly after having my bilateral mastectomy, I had the TRAM, had to have resurgery, because they tried to save the umbilical with the mesh. That herniated, so I had to go back in for surgery to have that fixed. [Vicky]

DISAPPOINTMENT WITH RECONSTRUCTION

Reconstruction is typically viewed as the "Achilles heel" of prophylactic mastectomy in the sense that unhappiness about PM tends to focus on a woman's feelings about how her reconstruction looks or feels. While many feel generally pleased, or feel that others admire the work their surgeon did, assessment of satisfaction with reconstruction is a difficult self-judgment for many women, since no reconstruction restores the way a woman looked before surgery nor does it restore the sensory input which is lost. It is striking, however, that whatever unhappiness there is about reconstruction seems to be most often experienced as "coming with the territory," a not surprising part of exchanging safety for beauty or familiarity.

The great unknown of PM with reconstruction is how the reconstructed breasts will actually look when all the surgeries are complete. It is an act of faith and trust when a woman asks a surgeon to make her "new" breasts. Descriptions and photographs are guides to what is possible, but how a particular woman's body responds, how much of an artist a particular plastic surgeon is, and what complications are encountered, all contribute to the final product. Women seemed to understand in varying degrees that the final product was an artistic unknown. Some women in our study seemed negatively shocked when the breasts were not as they thought they would be; others seemed to understand this process as more of an approximation to an ideal.

Well, in terms of the reconstruction, it didn't come out great. It's not perfect; it's not like you see the actresses with perfectly round breasts and no scars and the tissue just looks—well, not natural, but it doesn't look like it's been through multiple surgeries and things like that. So because of the incisions that I've had and puckering in some areas. My left breast was always a little bit bigger than my right breast; so when they put the same size implants in, there was a little bit extra tissue hanging around the nipple on the left, and it kind of caves in a little bit. It really—because they're subcutaneous, it's a big knot, really. They don't kind of fall in natural position. It's difficult to explain, but they really, you know.

When I move—yes, when I move, they kind of just stay right there. [Laughs] When the rest of my body moves. They will never sag. I was told that they will never sag. They're going to stay right there. But that also—it's great, if I'm not moving. But it does look unnatural, if I'm moving about. Only without clothes on. With clothes on, you really cannot tell. I've had many people tell me that they would have never guessed. Even in a bikini, you can't really tell, unless you see my scars. [Valerie]

Three years later, I'm still not finished [with the reconstruction]. So, that can give you an idea [of the problems] . . . I would choose the same [reconstruction] in a different way. Like maybe I need to know and understand better what I am getting into, who is doing it. I don't know. I had terrible confidence in the person doing it. I don't think I should have. I won't get into any more. . . . Well, it's an adjustment. They still don't feel comfortable. They never will, you know. It's not like, gee whiz, they removed the old ones, they put something underneath, and now I'm comfortable. No, it's not particularly comfortable, you know. I mean, over the past three years, I've gone from pain to uncomfortable to just comfortable. You know, you name it. With what I have right now . . . I'm moderately uncomfortable. I can live with it . . . It's either that or they both come out. But, you know, if I get under the knife again, it's remove them both. They're not worth it [the implants]. [Sonia]

Some women seem to take as a given the rhythm of surgeries comprising reconstruction with expanders and implants.

But, I think I was pleased that I had the reconstruction done, and I think that helped kind of ease the transition because I was still going in periodically to have my expanders filled and get to the right size and then having the surgery where my implants were actually put in. I think just kind of following through with all of that kind of helped. It was kind of a sense of rebuilding what had been lost, and that helped. So, I feel very much myself now with the implants, and it's been an okay transition, I'd say. [Irene]

Others women found it very difficult to have repeated surgeries.

Well, it's kind of bad because of all the surgeries and all the millions of times. I'm supposed to go back for a chest wall exam, and this summer I will. But like for a year, I felt like I needed to not go near the hospital, because I needed to stop being a patient for a while because it's not in the mastectomy, but the reconstruction, you go back for about a year. You keep going back. You've got to get your nipples done, and your nipples tattooed and on and on it goes . . . So, yes, the recovery was pretty intense, it was. I wouldn't lie to anybody if there was somebody who would feel better off without them. I mean I've read there are women that don't care about reconstruction, and if they don't, they're lucky because the reconstruction was what nearly killed me, you know. [Meredith]

Other women reported no problems with their breast reconstruction surgery.

Knock on wood, [there were] none. Yes, I mean, it was a amazing job [the reconstruction]. I'm sure he would say that, too [the plastic surgeon]. [Laughter] He'd be very proud of his work. [Beth]

SPORTS AND OTHER ACTIVITIES AFTER SURGERY

In thinking about what it means to get back to "normal," many women compare what they could do in terms of sports or physical exercise both before and after surgery.

[As far as playing sports, was that involved at all, affected at all?] Not as far as running. Swimming is different because you do stretch and pull, but it hasn't stopped me. I just know that I'm going to have some pain. Pretty much anything I do, though, you have to figure you're going to have some chest pain. That doesn't go away. Like if I shovel, if I rake, if I play baseball with my kids, if I swim. Hiking or something like that wouldn't do it. Waterskiing kills. I was a pretty avid water skier before, and I really don't do it that much anymore because it really does pull on your chest. It's four years later, and if I really touch my chest, it still hurts. It's still painful, and I'm beginning to think that that probably isn't going to go away. [Meredith]

Women in our study had a range of physical activity both presurgery and, of course, postsurgery. Some women, to whom exercise is important, could not do at least some of the sports they had previously enjoyed. They felt that giving them up was part of the price of surgery. Most of these women found other sports they could continue to do or took up postsurgery with their doctors' approval. Some countered their doctor's advice about physical activity. One woman attributed giving up exercising to surgery. And some women experienced no change in what they could do after their PM surgery.

Well, before my surgery—fortunately, this is probably the worst part—this is the worst thing my surgery did: I used to go to the gym six days a week. After my surgery, I tried to get back into it, and I never did. So that is probably an equal loss to my body parts, is my inability, really, to continue my exercise program. It was partially due to the sensations I was having. It was so uncomfortable to do things with my upper body for a good couple of months. Then I didn't have any stamina after that. My endurance was way down. I really haven't been able to regain that . . . I always do an hour on the treadmill, and I can't. I can do, like, five minutes and I'm wiped out. I can't breathe, I'm weak, I'm dizzy, I'm nauseous. So I'm very discouraged about that. It's been ten years, and I can't get back into an exercise program. [Valerie]

Oh, yes. I have trouble sitting for any length of time, especially straight up. I can't ride a bike like I used to. I can ride it, but I can't go very far. Walking is pretty easy, but anything where I have to sit or fold my body in any way, I have a problem. [Laura]

With the reconstruction, one side has been more successful than the other side. One side, movement is back to a 100 percent. The other side, I would say it's 90 or 95 percent. There is a way in which I can lift, if I lift my hands straight up over my head, with my right arm, it pulls, sort of a tugging across the chest, whereas that does not happen at all on the left side. Unfortunately, I'm a righty, so it doesn't feel comfortable to play tennis or something like that. [Sandra]

No, I do whatever I've always done. I'm just not as active. I'm a little bit older, but I'm more apprehensive about falling because of my stomach is not at a 100 percent because of the mesh. It just didn't do as well as I thought it was going to. But that, I think, is just me. [Vicky]

Many women felt they were able to return to their presurgery exercise programs following a period of reduced activity.

It hasn't [affected my ability to play sports] I think, initially, after the surgery, it took me a long time. I felt very tired for even several months. I think it took me a while to get kind of back on my feet. But, I'm sure that was a combination of surgery, having had a baby, going back to work, and a bunch of other things in terms of becoming active again. It took a little while for me to get jumpstarted, but I find I can do everything now I used to do. I run and I can still play golf when I can find time to do that and other things. So, it really hasn't hindered my activity at all [Irene].

Joyce, a yoga practitioner, had had problems after surgery using her arms in the ways she was used to doing as part of her yoga routine. She got a physical therapy consult and did exercises typically given to women who had had mastectomies. This helped to relax her shoulder, stomach, and neck muscles and she found the exercises very helpful. Joyce said she feels it would be helpful if such consults were routine for women following any type of mastectomy, as they would avoid some of the loss of mobility she had experienced.

REGRET ABOUT RECONSTRUCTION

Just as women's investment in their natural breasts varied considerably, so, too, did women's concern about the pleasing qualities of their reconstructed breasts. Some were quite disappointed and had various surgical adjustments made. Others lived more easily with the results, glad that they were still free of their natural breasts which had threatened their future well being. When there was great disappointment or when women who were disappointed later learned from family members or others about more successful forms of reconstruction, they did sometimes voice regret with the type of procedure they had chosen or, in one case, with the person they had trusted to do the reconstruction.

You said is there anything that we would do differently maybe, and that's the type of reconstruction I had. They tell you that they have other kinds that are more natural looking. I knew that at the time, but I just felt like it's just so difficult to go through that, and I didn't really have the time or that, you know, I didn't know if I could go through that at the time. But kind of, if I had, I'd have a better result right now, and I wish I had the result I would have had . . . Yes, I would have been had to be gone for weeks [if I had chosen the TRAM flap and had to go to Boston], and I just didn't have anybody to watch my kids for that long that I would have felt comfortable with. So I did this. But it's impacted me a lot, because that would have been more natural, I think. [Alice]

I would say that out of clothing, they certainly do not look like real breasts. For anybody to have the anticipation, the expectations that what they're going to get is going to replicate what they had before is unrealistic. I think that's really important to note because I think you have to—if you go into it, you have to know that what you're going to have is not—and I know most doctors, Dr. X, showed some very graphic photographs to give you an idea of what they're going to look like or what some people's have looked like and it's going to depend a lot on your body and how big you want to be.

I did one thing that could have been a mistake and I think—it was my choice and I will point this out. I think it's kind of important to note, it was that I wanted to be as big as I was before. Dr. X warned me that in doing so, he was going to have to really, really stretch me as far as those pectoral muscles would go and it was—there was a certain point where he said, "I can't really stretch you much more than this." In doing so, when he went and put in the implants, the skin is sewn back together and all was very, very, very taut. As a result down the line, my scar—my original scar which was just like a little hairline scar, which would have looked lovely as it faded with time, but what can happen with that—and what happened with me, was that I developed like a keloid . . . But then he had some patients who had them—you know, like one patient who had them for about ten years, and she was fine. He said, "But I can't guarantee you." I said, "Hey, if I can go five years without surgery, I'd be a happy camper." It's now been ten years. So I felt like this is all gravy for me. Plus having the actual implants put in and taken out is not that big of a deal of surgery. [Fay]

The only thing that I would change, like I said, is I would probably not have the TRAM, I would probably just have what my sister had the year after I had mine done, had a bilateral mastectomy and opted for just the silicone [implants] . . . I would only not have the TRAM. I think I would just have the breast implant. [Vicky]

I'm very satisfied, other than the nipples. Other than the nipples. Because, like I said, I can wear a bathing suit and you can't tell. They are very real looking, other than the nipples. That's my only thing I feel bad about. [Hanna]

Would I change anything? I would have asked them to make my nipples bigger and darker. I'm serious. It's the one thing that bugs me. I would have gained a little bit more weight so my second one could be better. I didn't have enough tissue to quite finish the second one right. [Meredith]

The reconstruction could use some work. But I'm not posing nude in any magazines or anything, so it's just a personal—it's really a personal feeling that I have about that. I don't know. As the years go by, I think, "Well, I'm too old to go back and have a little nip and tuck here." And to what end, you know? [Valerie]

REGRET: WOULD I HAVE ESCAPED CANCER WITHOUT IT?

Not one woman in our study said unequivocally that she felt she had made the wrong decision in having the prophylactic mastectomy. In fact, regret was in a few cases whispered; it was a brief comment but never a sweeping conclusion. Regret about the nature of the reconstruction which had been chosen or the choice of surgeon was occasionally expressed. What was more common was postsurgical wonder about whether the woman had truly needed to have the PM. Since some women from hereditary cancer families, even those with *BRCA1/2* mutations, do not get breast cancer, it is true that some of the women who had PM surgery might have escaped being diagnosed with breast cancer, even without surgery. The problem is that no one knows which women would have been part of this lucky cohort. Some women did think about this possibility after PM surgery, with some sadness or feeling approaching regret, as they contemplated if the surgery had been as critical as they had finally come to decide it was.

Yes, I do. I do wonder. There are times I don't know if I jumped the gun by doing it [having a PM]. On one avenue, it is nice to know that my chances, because I, basically, was told that there a 95 percent chance of me developing breast cancer at one point in my life, as opposed to being knocked to 1 to 4 percent, is what I was, basically, told. So, to me, those odds were much better. It was more favorable for me because my children are everything to me. So that's, basically, why I did what I did. I didn't like the odds that I had piled up against me. [Hanna]

Well, I've asked myself that a lot, and I'm not positive. I don't want to say I'm positive I did the right thing in the first place, because I'm not. I'm still here, so I'm glad. It's not that I go around regretting it. I don't. But deciding whether to do it again is, I couldn't be positive. I'd say probably 75 percent sure. So I didn't have the benefit of having that gene testing back then . . . Not for sure, right. I mean, I don't regret it, but I'm not positive. You know, I did something pretty big that impacted my husband and me a lot. Even though he never complains ever, it's still, I feel kind of bad for him. You know, I had to do this, and—I mean, he's been great but I know that I've done something that maybe wasn't necessary and look, you know. You know the society we live in, and he's given up a lot, and I feel bad.

I think maybe at first I was more sure, and now, you know, it's easier to think maybe nothing would have happened, you know. I'm not positive. I'm wondering, you know, if that just will change over my whole life. But, you know, lately I've been wondering, you know. But I don't know. So 75, 80 percent, I don't know. . . . Yes, it's just really hard, you know, deciding this out of nowhere except from family members. Well, I was wondering what, you know, what they would find? I didn't really have any idea, and that's kind of difficult, you know, to know that I did something this drastic with no idea. [Alice]

Occasionally, now, I get to feeling like should I have done it or should I not have? Especially, like I said, when people that are insensitive to issues, it makes you feel like, I don't know. You feel like you were you too hasty in making that decision, or should I have just waited and see what the cancer society is going to come up with. Then, again, when I sit down and rationally think about it, my kids were my drive. That is that. There were times when I said, "Oh, what it would be like to have a set of breasts again that you could feel." They're gone and I wish they were there, but they're not. So do I get upset over it and cry about it, you can't, because if you do, you do it all the time. To me, I can't do that. I have to focus and just say that I believe in my heart that I did the right thing. [Hanna]

Just because that's when they said the risk were beginning to really grow as you get in your thirties. I was getting in my thirties. I was twenty-nine. We discussed that if we were going to do it, that we should do it. I had a cousin that had gotten it [breast cancer] at twenty-eight. My father's cousin had gotten breast cancer at twenty-eight. We just felt that—I feel now that maybe we acted kind of like out of a panic, that maybe we could have waited. It wasn't like—it didn't have to be so rushed. Not that I feel like I made the wrong decision, but I feel like sometimes when you get drastic news like that, you work out of like a panic. I feel like we did kind of. Part of the decision was based on that like panic that we've got to do it because—not that it's the wrong thing. Not that I'm saying we should have waited a long time, but I feel like maybe it didn't have to be as rushed as it was.

I didn't get reconstruction. I feel a little bit regret for that now. Like I feel maybe if I were to do it again, that I would consider that more . . . Any regrets? Regret, yes, sometimes. There are times I have in mind, "I wish I didn't do this." But if I had to really like sit down and really discuss it out, I would say that I would do it again. I really think I would do it again. But there are times, there many times, that I feel I never should have done this. . . . [Harriet]

Well, now that I'm talking to you, I regret I didn't seek out individual counseling before because of how things went and even though I was all tapped out with other sorts of counseling. I'm thinking I probably should have brought [up] a lot of my personal feelings about it. [Valerie]

Such reflection among the women we interviewed leads to thinking about what might have made the experience of prophylactic mastectomy easier for these women. This topic we will consider in the next chapter.

CHAPTER 9

What Would Have Helped?

We asked women in our study about what might have helped them with their prophylactic mastectomy experience. In particular, we asked if they had the opportunity to talk to someone who had previously undergone mastectomy, especially prophylactic mastectomy and, if this discussion was helpful. We also asked if emotional support from a psychologist seeing them individually, or as a couple, or in a group would have been useful. In answering these questions, women revealed more about their PM experience to us. What became increasingly clear was that PM was a challenging, difficult experience for many, but one which left most women feeling very satisfied overall with the difficult choice they had made. We will look at more of those satisfactions in Chapter 10.

PEER SUPPORT FROM WOMEN WHO HAD BEEN THROUGH PM

A major tenet of this book is that women making decisions about PM, preparing for surgery, or adjusting after surgery could be tremendously helped by learning about what this rare and, what some call "radical," experience has been like for others. From these stories, women can learn how those who have a PM feel about their choices, and what proved to be important to them. Such information is not very easy to come by in the general population or even in medical circles. In such circumstances, social support research suggests that the guidance of others who have already walked this path—"peers"—as they are called in such research, is invaluable, very reassuring, and informative to patients with a wide range of conditions.[1, 2, 3] How else does a woman know what to expect from this surgery, what is expected during recovery, and what is atypical of the surgery? Only the stories of other women can answer these questions.

> [Women] who are at the same level you are, who are maybe going into it [PM] or have just gone through it . . . I think it would have been very helpful for me to find another human being who was going through this, because, again, to me there was so much of the feeling of I'm outside the realm of normal life. And to normalize this experience by connecting you with others, I think, would be incredibly valuable. [Sandra]

As many women in our study commented, no matter how available surgeons and plastic surgeons were to them, they did not actually know what a woman's chest feels like after PM surgery. Nor would they know how it feels to find oneself without breasts, to go through a long process of reconstruction, or to wonder, in a communal dressing room, if they should take off their shirt in public.

> I think they [women deciding about PM] would have to draw on some experience maybe of somebody else. You really don't know. I wasn't prepared for physical feelings or emotional feelings, so you have to really explore and think about what they've heard other women experience and think, "Is that an issue for me? How would I react?" [Valerie]

A considerable number of women in our study had been able to talk to someone who had previously undergone PM. Those who had this experience offered some caution about such discussions. First, because of the relative rarity of PM versus mastectomies done for cancer, in a number of cases, the women considering PM were given the names of women who had undergone mastectomy for cancer. This experience proved to not be so useful and, in at least one case, was described as being rather burdensome to be in what the woman felt was a primarily unequal circumstance.

> I had the Breast Cancer Society send me a patient advocate, and she was very helpful in telling me that she had had reconstruction, you know, what the recovery was going to be like. So I knew. During the recovery she was good with vitamin supplements and things that

the doctor wouldn't tell me about, the different pains and things that you have. But it was kind of weird because I felt like I was kind of lucky because I don't have breast cancer and she actually had it recur in another breast and she wasn't doing that well. So I felt kind of funny getting help from her. You know what I mean? I felt like I should be helping her, but she was very helpful. [Meredith]

While the surgery may be the same, the emotions of recovery under these two different conditions appear to be quite dissimilar. For the women with cancer, there are many frightening experiences ahead, many looming larger than the surgery they had undergone. In some cases, they had had strong medical advice that mastectomy was the correct treatment for their cancer; in other cases, they might have had a choice between lumpectomy and mastectomy and had made this choice themselves. But in either case, the emphasis was on reducing the cancer burden and there was considerable fear both about the extent of cancer found during surgery and the extent to which it had been removed by surgery.

For women deciding about PM, the ultimate goal is also to defeat cancer, but to defeat it before it actually occurs. The decision is a highly cerebral one, weighing risks and benefits which are abstract and do not consider existing, growing cells threatening to take over a woman's life. The questions are largely quality of life decisions, about how this surgical method of, hopefully, avoiding cancer will affect one's self-image, sexuality, and relationships in the long run. Thus, women who were given names of others who had undergone mastectomy for cancer were grateful for their time and attention, but did not find the interaction and information as useful as did the women who talked to others who had undergone truly *prophylactic* mastectomy. Women whose doctors did not guide them to peers or who were not resourceful in calling the American Cancer Society or a breast cancer organization found it difficult to locate women who had undergone a PM. In some cases, women were given lists of previous PM patients by their surgeons. This was found to be very helpful and women had often contacted one or more women on the list. They did voice worries that the women who were on the lists were possibly the most satisfied in the doctor's practice, and not a random sample, so that they were perhaps not hearing from the less satisfied customers. Nonetheless, women heard some range of response from the previous patients whose names the doctors had given them and they used their discussions to make the "Is this an issue for me?" comparison.

Right, to know, God, what does it feel like? [not to have breasts] … What can you physically do after the surgery, and how am I going to feel physically and all of that. That was very, very helpful and very interesting because the first woman I spoke to sort of painted a kind of bleak picture for me of how she felt afterwards and went on and on in this sort of negative vein, but ultimately said at the end of the conversation, "But I'm really glad I did it," and I thought, wow. She sounded so negative about not having, you know, energy, [she] couldn't move and couldn't do, and would get up, put her makeup—, a month later would still get up in the morning, put on makeup and get back in bed.

But then the next woman I talked to was playing tennis within four weeks of her surgery and with more, I think, you know, her attitude was much closer to what mine is like and would probably be, and she painted a wonderful picture of the whole thing for me, and a very honest one, lots of neat little tips. I just found speaking with those women more helpful than about anything else. [Fay]

I most wanted to know like her husband's reaction. I was very scared about the surgery, obviously. I didn't know what that was going to be like, how much pain and that sort of thing. [Kate]

In retrospect, some women who had not spoken to a peer said they would have found it useful to talk to a peer counselor as they recalled the difficulties of the PM experience.

No, I didn't [talk to someone who had a PM]. I probably should have. I would suggest a woman to do that, but I did not. Because, I mean, it is a very hard thing to go through. I think only someone in the same boat can really help you, you know, tell you feelings about it. You know, to discuss how you're going to feel about the different things you go through afterwards. So, I did not talk to somebody, but I probably—I feel like it's probably the right thing to do. [Harriet]

I wish I could have talked to someone. I know it sounds like I talked to a lot of medical people, but I wish I had—I guess I didn't get all the information I wanted. I wish I had known … But, no, I think you're never going to have all the information you want. I thought I had it covered—God, I think I talked to every doctor under the sun. [Julia]

FAMILY EXEMPLARS–PROS AND CONS

Some women in our study had family members who preceded them in undergoing prophylactic mastectomy and this was very useful in some cases. One woman said her sisters could not really provide support for her since she was worried about them (often this was because the sister had undergone a mastectomy for cancer) and thus, could not get support from them for her surgery.

When a sister or other close relative had previously undergone PM and they were confidantes, this was typically very helpful for both women in that it made it easier to broach rather intimate questions.

But, again, I think I had my own kind of support network built in with having two sisters who had now gone through this and having been put in contact with another young woman who had been through it. I think having so many people to talk to about it, as much as I needed to, really, I think, kind of filled what otherwise might have been a gap for me in having somebody to talk to. [Irene]

A proviso, of course, is that sisters, even close sisters, are not always at ease in discussing intimate details of their lives. Also, sibling rivalry can come into play about whose experience was the best or worst, whose doctor was better, whose reconstructed breasts are more attractive, who was stronger and braver, or had the most support. Also, sisters, to be helpful to one another, have to allow room for the other to make different decisions about how they approach and deal with PM surgery. They may opt for different reconstruction techniques, different doctors, and/or different approaches to physical activity following surgery. While it is usually interesting and valuable to hear of sister's PM experience, few questions are asked if a judgmental attitude guides the response.

On the contrary, trust in known family relationships may lead even women who consider themselves quite independent to do what others in the family believe is best.

Then I found out that a cousin of mine had just had a prophylactic mastectomy. A bilateral. She is not related to me by blood. My cousins called me and said, "C's had a prophylactic mastectomy. You might want to talk to her." So I called her up, and I said, "Okay, what did you do?" She told me.

I said [to my cousin with the PM], "How did you decide what procedure to have?" She said, "Well, I really left it all up to my brother because I was in [another continent], and he arranged everything. He was the one who decided." I thought, "Well, if he's a surgeon and he decided that this is what's best for his sister and she's about my size, then he's confirming my view," which was, guess what, for little [i.e. small-breasted] people, this is probably it. Doing another route is probably not going to be compatible with a high quality of life. . . . It was a wonderful thing that that happened, for me, because it meant that I had somebody who was close to me that I could speak to about her personal experience with this and about the decision that she had made. [Joyce]

NOT FOR EVERYONE

As with all forms of social support, talking with a peer was not for everyone. Some women in our study simply felt that they did not need to talk to someone else, that they had made up their mind about the procedure and that was all they needed to know.

IS THERE LIFE AFTER PM?

One woman eloquently described what she received from talking to a peer was the fundamental reassurance that one survived the PM surgery, that it came not to be on the "front burner" but the "back burner," and that life eventually came to have other foci after the procedure. This advice is was what she most wanted to hear from a true "expert."

I think the most helpful thing psychologically is for a woman to speak to somebody else who's done it and [who] tells you, "Guess what, there's life at the end of this. You're going to grow into your new boobs, and you're going to forget that you've got them." [Joyce]

PSYCHOLOGICAL SUPPORT

While about half of the women in our study had at some point in their lives seen a psychologist or therapist, only three saw a psychologist or therapist before surgery to discuss their decision about PM. A few women sought psychological treatment after surgery.

> Just everything in general with it, with the decision, with the aftereffects, the way your body feels. I did end up into counseling afterwards. I did seek out a therapist to talk to regarding it. Basically, I came to terms with it when she said to me, "Well, basically, who has a perfect body?" When I looked, and I sat and I thought, I said, "Well, yes, that's true." Because she said, "As a woman, we always want to have something we don't have. Some of us want a flat stomach, some of us want bigger thighs, some of us want smaller breasts or bigger breasts." She said, "None of us are ever really happy with what we have. So what is the perfect body? Describe it." I couldn't do it, so, therefore, I came to terms with it. Really, none of us do have perfect bodies, and we always want what we can't have. [Hanna]

The majority of women in the study did not have psychological counseling, but many of these women advocated for the availability of psychological services for women both before and after surgery.

> I think it [psychological counseling] is very useful. For people, it's an emotional decision to make. It's a decision that is based on sort of medical evidence, because most people I think who are going to think about doing a prophylactic surgery have suffered trauma and loss and have grieved probably the loss or the close loss or close death of loved ones, and there's a tremendous amount of fear and anxiety. So, I do think, yes, it would be very helpful. [Sandra]

Some women talked about their usual resistance to therapy or support groups, but said that they felt, at least retrospectively, that the situation of undergoing PM was different, that this was a circumstance where psychological support would have been very helpful.

> I think that it would be useful for most people. I think that it wouldn't have hurt me at all. I tend to be my own psychologist. [Laughs] I didn't want to, like, go—I was offered, you know, to go afterwards, like, to have—go to like a support group or whatever for women who had breasts removed, but I didn't do that, for a whole bunch of reasons. But I just didn't really feel a need

to. But I think that it would be a nice component. I think there's a lot of—I think there are a lot of fears and questions that any woman is going to have about it about how—like, I think it would have been nice to have been able to ask somebody, "What about this expectation that I have of myself to do well with this afterwards and then what if I wake up and I'm wrong about myself and I'm, like, devastated?" [Fay]

Well, I think they would have hopefully made me think of the future and probably look at every facet in the future and examine what the possibilities might be. I didn't really have an opportunity to think, "Well, what's this going to do to my marriage? What's this going to do to my physical health?" [Valerie]

Yes, I think that probably would have been helpful. The truth is, at the time I probably would have said, "I don't need it, and I don't want it." But looking back on it, I think, you know, I was like a little, you know—I don't know if you can ever prepare yourself for such a thing, but I would have liked to have been a little more prepared. [Harriet]

The theme of wanting help for feelings of loss and grief after the prophylactic mastectomy was a common one within our cohort.

I thought it would have been great. Now. At the time, I don't know if I would have went through with it, but at this time, I think everybody should prior to going into it only because if I had known some of the feelings such as the comments that the doctor made to me of how many of us do have a perfect body, I think that that may have helped me through the depression that I suffered afterwards. I think it would have helped me better, and I probably wouldn't have been so like, boom, because you do have like a sense of loss and grief. You really do go through a grieving process, like say six months to a year after you've had this done. At least that's the way it was with me. I felt that I really lost something. I didn't at that time feel whole. It took me a while to feel whole again, but now I feel complete so I'm fine. But there was a time that I did not feel complete. [Hanna]

I think, yes, because I didn't do it, and I think it would have been nice because I don't bare myself. Maybe other people have support. I'm kind of an island, and for me it would have been really nice besides my husband. You know, when you're talking to your family members, they love you, and I think they want to tell you what you want to hear and they're protective. And your friends can be protective . . . It really would have been nice to talk to somebody objective. [Julia]

Some women felt psychological consultations would have helped them recognize the extent of the emotional problems they faced post-surgery.

I think so, because I think I would have identified my anxiety and depression earlier. I think that might have helped me get to a decision earlier. Because, had somebody asked me questions like, "Are you having trouble focusing? Are you having trouble sleeping?"when I looked at the list and realized that things like gingivitis were classic signs of chronic depression, and I realized that I had these . . . I think I'd probably have done the surgery a year and a half before. So, yes, in the end, I think that. If you're talking that, that's what I would be specifically looking for. I'd be looking for low-level grades of anxiety and depression in people, because you can pretend about it, but then it's not there for a little while, but then it comes creeping back in.

What prevented me from doing that? I think the fact that I didn't realize that I was suffering from anything, from any psychological consequences. I think it was just that I didn't realize that I had depression, and so I didn't think I needed psychological services. I got every other kind of service you can imagine. If it was one thing that was missing on my palette of services that I hadn't found to myself and it wasn't offered to me, it would have been that. As I say, had I realized I was depressed, maybe I would have asked for it. [Joyce]

CHARACTERISTICS OF THE PSYCHOLOGIST

It was important to the women in the study that a psychologist helping women with PM-related issues was informed about prophylactic mastectomy, about the reasons why women undergo PM, about types of reconstruction, and about the complications and side effects of such surgery. Women were seeking empathy and even voiced a wish that a psychologist working with women considering or adapting to PM would ideally have undergone PM herself.

> Yes. And I think it would have been really helpful to have had somebody as the counselor who had gone through it. [Laura]

On the other hand, they did not want to talk to a psychologist who had fixed ideas about PM, but rather with someone who would help them express their own feelings about the surgery. Someone who would try to discover if the match with what the surgery offered was a good one in their case.

Some women talked about things that would be barriers to receiving counseling. Often, it was the recognition that the emotional aspects of the surgery were frightening. Women talked about how little they had let themselves think about their emotions as they made a largely intellectual decision about the pros and cons of PM. Other women spoke about availability of having a psychologist associated with the medical clinic where they were already going to see the surgeons, oncologists, and plastic surgeons, which would minimize the barrier of having to find one on their own. Some talked also about the barrier of available time for these additional appointments.

> I think probably the only thing that might have prevented me from doing it was just [finding] time for yet another doctor's appointment. [Irene]

Scheduling ease for psychologist appointments was important.

> I think I would have liked people available for me when I needed it . . . More like just mental health counseling where I could call up and say, "I need to talk to somebody today," or "I need to schedule an appointment for next Wednesday." [Laura]

Other women felt just the assurance that a mental health professional whom they had met would be available when needed would have been helpful to them.

> I would think if somebody had come back and had given me a card and said, "If you have any questions, you know my number, I'm available if you need to talk," I think that that would make a lot of people feel a little bit more relieved because they don't know how they're going to be [after the PM]. [Janice]

Some women talked about how having psychological consultation "built into" the presurgical workup would have been preferable to feeling that they were being referred to a psychologist because someone thought they were having problems or were psychologically unstable.

> Because if they didn't say it [the psychological consultation] was a standard part of it, I might be offended. If they say, "We're going to send you for a blood test to make sure you're all right, a psychologist, a urinalysis . . . " and the psychologist is on the list of things, then I think you just blow it off and say, "Fine." [Joyce]

Support groups were mentioned by some women as a desired way to meet other women in similar medical circumstances. Again, it was voiced that it would be important for the group to be just for women who had undergone PM without having had a cancer diagnosis. While there were often support groups for cancer patients who had mastectomies, women with cancer were thought to be in substantially different (and more fear-inducing) circumstances than those of the women who had undergone PM. The differences were such that mixing women whose surgeries might have been similar, but whose cancer status was different, was clearly not advisable.

> I wish there was some kind of a support group for women who have gone. Like [the group] "Why Me" is for those with cancer. I wish there was a support group for women who have gone through this and didn't have cancer. [Laura]

> I do think for women who do have prophylactic mastectomies, if there was a group of people that talked that didn't have cancer, I think that would be helpful I mean because you don't fit in with the cancer group. [Julia]

There were some women whom we interviewed who simply did not feel they needed psychological help during this time in their lives. In some cases, this was because they were not having major emotional problems or because they were so independent as to find it uncomfortable to think about talking with someone about their concerns about PM. Other women felt that their family and friends "filled the bill" in terms of their mental support needs.

> I don't know. Yes. Yes, if there were issues [about the PM]. By then it's all over with, and there's really nothing to deal with. Like your

body's getting better, but I think your emotions are healed at that point. I don't think there was any trauma afterwards to get over. At least, in my case, like I said I was so relieved and elated that I was anxious to tell people. That was my reaction. [Kate]

[Did you want to talk to other women who had undergone PM?] No, I don't think it probably would have made any difference. I'm kind of an independent cuss ... No, not really, not with me being the way I am. Like I say, I can see where some people, like my cousin, it was really helpful to her to have somebody to talk to that had been through that, and I know with patients and stuff that some people are like that. But with me, I don't think it would have made any difference. [Emily]

I think when you start telling people they need to see a counselor and talk about it, I think you make them have different feelings. I think you bring upon that there's something that I'm doing that's not correct, so I need to go talk to someone ... I think they're making it a negative thing, that you should be feeling these things, you should be uncomfortable, you should be—your husband's not going to, you know, love you anymore if you need to go to a [counselor] —I think if you and your husband decide on your own that you'd like to go see somebody, I think that's great. But when you start suggesting all these things and that they should be [unclear]—then they're going to be thinking that way. And if they don't need it, they're going to think they're even worse off. I'm supposed to be having these feelings, and I'm not. [Chantal]

I'm Irish. It wouldn't have helped .... I don't like anybody inside my head. I would have balked. I would have balked for my own self. I would have balked out of what feelings I had towards a psychologist. [Ingrid]

The additional cost for mental health treatment was thought to possibly be a barrier for about a third of the study group. However, many women had health insurance and others felt that the type of brief consultation they might have sought would not be too expensive and might have been helpful to them in making decisions about the major, life-altering surgery they were considering at the time.

In general, women retrospectively felt that avenues of psychological support should be available to women considering PM. Many wished they had taken advantage of or been offered some form of psychological support before surgery and wished that there was an easy way to find appropriate psychological treatment following surgery, if desired. They seemed to indicate that a woman did not have to doubt her motives for it to be valuable to review and test them before surgery and that it also would be valuable to try to anticipate the changes surgery would bring before making a final decision. Once surgery was accomplished, many women thought that psychological counseling could help normalize the feelings women experienced and provide support through the "rough spots." Some also felt that they had diagnosable psychological conditions (e.g., depression) and that seeing a psychologist might have speeded up getting appropriate treatment and hence, helped them to feel better sooner.

Peer relationships were invaluable to many women in the study. Given the degree to which PM is relatively rare and the range of reactions to it which can occur, it was enormously helpful for some of our cohort to talk to women who had undergone the experience. In some ways, this emotionally trumped the value accorded to even good medical advice, as it spoke to and answered women's darkest fears about disfigurement, sexual attractiveness, and pain. It was also living proof that one could get beyond all the planning and worrying and find satisfaction and peace in a life without one's natural breasts.

However, in both instances—psychological support and talking with peers—it was crucial that the help be targeted specifically to women without cancer. Talking to cancer patients as peers who had undergone mastectomies or who had undergone prophylactic mastectomies on their healthy remaining breast was not regarded as very helpful and was sometimes described as burdensome and awkward. Women who were considering PM who had not had cancer found it very difficult to talk with cancer patients and did not feel that their decision making process was similar to those made by women who had cancer. It also made them feel guilty since they were not immediately worrying about cancer treatment and survival. Support groups also needed to be solely for women without cancer who were considering or had undergone PM. When these groups were mixed or where the woman was the only non-cancer patient in the group, she reported that this experience was neither helpful nor comfortable.

Given the relative rarity of prophylactic mastectomy, it may be difficult to find a support group solely for women without cancer.

However, new technological advances which make possible online, Skype, MegaMeeting, or other visual computer linkages may also make possible the creation of support groups where women from different centers could be combined into a single, useful group setting. Sharing thoughts and feelings about PM, the reactions of family and friends, and descriptions of postsurgical symptoms may help women feel less alone and more prepared for this significant life change.

CHAPTER 10

What Was Gained: Satisfactions

Women in our study who had undergone bilateral prophylactic mastectomy (PM) in the absence of cancer were extremely articulate and exuberant about what they had gained from undergoing this surgery. We asked them what they thought would be different now in their lives if they had not had surgery and what they felt were the benefits of this surgery.

RELIEF: "I SAVED MY OWN LIFE"

Almost all the women in our group were very clear that they felt deep relief at having undergone this surgery; they spoke of being "elated." They felt it was likely that, had they not had surgery, they might already have developed breast cancer or would be very worried about that prospect. They imagined that they would by now have had other breast biopsies and maybe other masses would have been found, if not outright, frightening breast cancer. Some women said they thought they might be dead by now without having undergone the surgery. The extent to which the cancer fears had intruded into their lives was perhaps clearer in their answers to this question than earlier in the interview.

> [If you did not have PM?] Oh, well, I think, certainly, I think I'd still be living with just kind of a constant nagging fear of when is it going to happen to me. I don't have that, certainly not on a day-to-day basis. I don't have that anxiety anymore. [Irene]

Still, I really am glad that I did it, because it's scary to know with all of the problems that I had prior to going through the surgery . . . I felt like I was given a death sentence and it was just a matter of time . . . [If you did not have a PM?] I'd probably be worrying all the time if I have cancer. Or then, again, I probably would have had cancer by now . . . On that note, I feel that I beat it in one way, because it is a scary thing . . . I worry at times. But I'm not like I used to be. It just doesn't consume my day and it doesn't consume the month, either. [Hanna]

It would be very different [if I didn't have PM]. I probably would be dead. That's what I was told.[Sonia]

I haven't changed my mind at all as to whether I should or shouldn't have had that. . . . I think if I didn't have this done, I would have cancer. [Laura]

I thought it was just going to be something I maybe was embarrassed about or just quiet about it, it's a personal thing. But I felt so good afterwards, and very quickly. . . . [If did not have PM surgery] I keep thinking I could have cancer, that kind of thing. Still going every six months, still doing the monthly exam, which was very nerve-racking to me, just scared me to death. Once every month having to think about that. Every time I came across an article about cancer I would sit there and read it. If there was a number to call, I'd cut it out if I needed it. Almost like a weird obsession, it was just such a part of my life. I don't have any of that now. [Kate]

"SAFE WITHIN MY OWN BODY"

Women's relationships to their bodies had clearly undergone change in many positive respects by the active steps they took through PM surgery to reduce their breast cancer risk. Some women also expressed relief that no cancer had been found in their breast tissue when it was examined postsurgery.

I feel like it's no longer this thing that's going to bail on me or betray me. It's an odd thing to think about your body, but I don't feel that about it anymore. [Kate]

I didn't feel safe within my own body. Having the bilateral mastectomies removed that fear. I mean it literally solved my problems. [Sandra]

HOW MUCH BETTER OFF?

The extent to which their breast cancer risks had been reduced was expressed differently by different women. When numbers were attached to this risk reduction, they varied from 80 percent to 100 percent. Women clearly understood that they were much safer now, at least statistically, than they have been before PM surgery. Some also spoke of their postsurgical period in relative terms, as being able to turn back time and fear to "normal" worry about population level breast cancer risk.

> I came back to a position where I probably was about as afraid of breast cancer as I was before my mother got it and I didn't know anything about it. [Kristen]
>
> Now [after the surgery], I really don't—I don't think of it [breast cancer] as often. I think of it just probably just once a month, when I get my period, and what's left of the breast is sore. [Valerie]
>
> I really don't feel like I'm going to get breast cancer, you know? I feel like that the studies that have come out since have said I'm not going to get it, you know, most likely, so, you know, 90-something percent change or whatever. So I really feel like I've dodged that bullet [because I got the PM] . . . so I worry less having had it. So I guess that's pretty great because I pretty much don't worry about it now. [Alice]
>
> No, I mean, some people think they need to have it done, but I think they may get talked into it because of family history. This was a family history situation, but I could have decided, as my sisters did, not to and just been more aggressive with mammograms. I just didn't want to be going that route, finding out every six months, I've got another cyst, and they've got to remove that one. I didn't want to go that route. I'd already had that done twice. It was more than enough. [Vicky]

When asked to evaluate the overall experience of having undergone prophylactic mastectomy, the women were usually lavish in their praise and clear about the high level of satisfaction they felt with the results. These were women who had put much thought into this decision to undergo a bilateral PM and had, in some cases, researched the surgery over a number of years. They were relieved when it was done, and felt it did very significantly reduce their worry about breast cancer. Even if the cosmetic result was not perfect, most women felt that PM had been a valuable experience of conquering fear of cancer.

> Ten, honestly [rated satisfaction on a scale of one to ten]. [Sandra]
>
> On a scale of one to ten, I'm going to say a ten, because I think if I went back to do it now, I don't think I'd change a single thing. [Joyce]
>
> Extremely satisfied. I really don't have any complaints about the support I've gotten from physicians, family, everybody. It's been a good process. [Irene]
>
> Yes, because the mastectomy, I'm a hundred percent. I can't imagine having done it any way else unless there was a cure. [Laura]
>
> I guess I'm satisfied in that I don't worry about—I hate to even say this, because maybe I should be. But I don't worry now about getting breast cancer so much. I feel like I did reduce my risk. [Harriet]
>
> I'm very happy [with the decision to have PM]. [Janice]

For some women, it seemed difficult many years after the PM surgery to express the deep vulnerability which they had experienced when they were sure that, without the surgery, they would get breast cancer. This was unsettling, but apparently did little to change the women's beliefs that they had made the right choice. Alice talked about this.

> Today I was thinking I would say 75 percent. You know, maybe that's not enough, you know, because I'm here. Did I really believe I wouldn't be? My husband thinks I believed I wouldn't be here, you know, and I don't know what I thought. So maybe it's 80 percent. I don't know. [Alice]

The high level of satisfaction which women experienced in their lives after PM led one woman to wish doctors would be more prescriptive in strongly recommending PM to women at high risk for breast cancer.

> Very satisfied with that. I think there should be more education. I think it should be supported more to do what I did. And like I said, the studies that came out that it really does have benefit didn't happen until after and for all I know they do advocate it

more. I just think there should be more support towards women who are high risk towards doing it. From the medical staff, who kind of leaves it up to> [you], and it is kind of an agonizing decision because they don't come right out and say, "Well, you know, we think you should." [Meredith]

RELIEF FROM DEPRESSION

The relief many of these women in our study felt after PM was also about not having the psychological burden of feeling at risk, which was described in heightened terms as they recalled how disturbed they had felt by their worry about breast cancer. Other women talked about feeling that they had stopped a family pattern which had gone on for generations, that they had defused the "time bomb" they felt inside themselves, and that a "cloud" they had not realized was there was lifted from their lives. What had felt like the inevitability of breast cancer had been stopped and this had major psychological effects for them.

[If had not had PM?] I think I might be dead. Or a real total head case. Because I'd still be worrying every time I had another lump. [Fay]

Now that I've had the surgery, I actually plan for the future more than I used to. I pretty much didn't plan too much for the future before that.... If I hadn't chosen to have it? Well, every single day, I'd be checking my breasts and wondering if today's the day. I wouldn't be able to sleep. I'd figure my life isn't going to be a long one. You'd think I'd be traumatized by having this, but I actually feel as if a cloud was lifted that I never knew that I had over me, like I suddenly feel I have a new lease on life because I actually might get to be an old lady. I have to put away more money for my retirement, but I had a cloud over my head that I had had since I was kid, so I didn't even know I had it I was so used to having it.

This feeling that I am going to get breast cancer, that my father probably will bury me. My mom was only fifty-six when she died, you know. My grandmother was fifty-one. Her mother was forty-three. So I would still be living that way, day to day, figuring who cares about tomorrow, not being able to sleep.... I used to wake up in a cold sweat thinking, "Oh, my God, I'm going to get this and my kids are so little." I used to feel there was a time bomb clicking inside my chest, and now I don't. . . . I feel I'm happier now than before I did it. So for me that's the positive thing. So that's why the tradeoff is, yes, I've got kind of funny-looking boobs, but I'm not pushing up daisies either. [Meredith]

No, I barely worry about it [breast cancer]. In some moments of sort of weakness and pain, I think, "Oh, my God, what if I'm the one in a million that," you know, so it's not completely eliminated. But it has been reduced to an almost insignificant amount. I still get checked. . . . I follow up very carefully on my health. But I was worried that I was going to end up sort of nonfunctional because my stress level was so high. [Sandra]

CONFIDENCE

A sense of confidence and trust in one's ability to make good decisions was a surprising postsurgical consequence for some women in the study.

Because as I say, I think—and this is the other benefit which relates to this—the other benefit that I had not counted on—this is probably a biggie—is that who knew that you could get through something like this with such flying colors? So because of that, I think it gave me a sense of self-confidence that I didn't otherwise have, to that extent, a sense of accomplishment. You know, and a sense of, "Well, if I can get through something like that and change some of my values and, you know, take charge of my life and do this thing and learn a lot about my health and know what needs to be done and do it, and do it with great bravado, that you feel like such a much better person." It really actually has given me something in terms of how I feel about myself, that I never would have had otherwise. So that was a terrific benefit. Plus, I also have—the icing on the cake with that is that now I am on referral lists. Now I get to participate in a study like this. It makes you feel like you have some—your life really has had a purpose. [Fay]

GAINS

Our women study participants talked about feeling they had gained time, "an incredible sense of peace," the possibility they would live to be an old lady, to be able to know their grandchildren, to be able to retire, and to retain the normal order and expectations most people have of their lives and potential lifespan. These were not small gains, but large ones in their eyes. The gains were not without cost, but what had been achieved seemed overwhelmingly more valuable than that which had been lost.

As I once told someone recently, I said, "You know what? If I had my whole life to live over—." And I know this sounds really crazy, "but I would not want to have missed out on every bit of what I went through in terms of my health with all this stuff." I said, "Because I learned so many lessons from it" . . . I had a certain appreciation of life, and have—to live every day to the fullest in a way that—I guess I was faced with my own mortality at a young age. I wouldn't take that lesson back for anything. So I'd go through every little bit that I went through just to be where I am right now; and I wouldn't trade places with anybody in terms of that. So I think it all happened for a reason . . . [Any regrets?] No, that was it. It was just a resounding no! [Laughs] [Fay]

I don't feel the pressure of having that cancer thing hanging over my head. I think I enjoy my life better. I think I'm more relaxed in the big scheme of things. I always felt before that it could happen any day, I've got to live my life right now, kind of feeling. This could be my last Christmas. Every time I went in to get a mammogram, it was like, this could be the last. So I'm much more relaxed now about things. . . . I actually see myself like being with my kids' children at some point in my life, and I never thought that way before. I never thought I would live that long to see my grandchildren. Obviously, my mom didn't, my dad didn't, and that cancer thing, boy, it really is pretty powerful. [Kate]

WOULD I DO IT AGAIN?

The many real-life decisions necessary to undergo a PM and to take the many steps to recovery may obscure the finality of the changes surgery brings. Dawning recognition of the losses involved and their finality, however, did not spawn regret.

I'm fine with it. Again, I wish there was sensation, more sensation than what's there, but there's not. So I guess there's good and bads [sic] to every decision we do. Again, they're only breasts, and it's not me. [Hanna]

The evolution of feelings is that you come to the reality that this is forever, so that's a little ... At some point, you realize that this is forever, you know, you have to deal with, you're never going to have that, and, at one point, I remember it hitting me like that this is forever. And it was difficult. I don't remember where along the line it was. But in the beginning, you kind of feel like, I don't know. It doesn't feel like a—I can't explain it. But you kind of feel like, okay, you had something that happened, but it's going to be okay. Then at some point it hits you, like, this is forever, and it's difficult. ... Yes, there are times when you just feel emotionally like, oh, I miss it. But if I had to sit down and actually say here what I would do, I would do it again. [Harriet]

SATISFACTIONS

In our group of women who chose prophylactic mastectomy, as well as in others studied in the medical literature,[1, 2] there is a high degree of satisfaction and a lack of regret in their decision to have the surgery. Listening to what women say, in the end, about their satisfaction, and their overall assessment of how they feel about what they chose to do can be informative and motivational for women making this decision. Hence, we have included many of their statements here to illustrate their feelings of euphoric (or sometimes less euphoric, but still positive) completion and relief.

I felt, like I said to Dr. X, the psychiatrist, before the surgery, one of the most important things that I felt was that this surgery—she told me, she made it very clear to me that the surgery's not 100 percent guaranteed. But I told her, I said, "You know, if fate happens to come along, and I do get breast cancer down the line by some fluke, I will never be able to say to myself that I didn't do everything I could have possibly done to help myself," like, to the point of having surgery. I still feel that way. You know, I just check regularly, but if it ever happens, you know, that's that thing. I did everything I could possibly do. I have absolutely no regrets, none ... I'm very glad I had it done. I mean, I can honestly say that I have never ever regretted it. [Kristen]

In terms of appearance and in terms of my, what my outcome might be, I'm satisfied with my decision. [Valerie]

I mean I think it's just kind of a day-by-day thing, and I've just kind of accepted that that's the way it is and [I] know that I can live with that because the alternative was this almost certainty that I would be facing a cancer diagnosis at some point. I think it was worth the tradeoff. That's how I view it...I would have to say even if I didn't have children, I would have had it done, because just watching, having had family members go through the process of getting diagnosed with cancer and then the treatment. It's a horrible ordeal and even when you catch it early, there's still no guarantee that you can beat it.

I think having, if you know that you have a real high risk because of your family history or whatever, I think this surgery is a real option for people. It certainly has made me feel much better about my prospects for living a long life and stuff, I'm sure... [Any regrets?] No, none. I'd do it again tomorrow if I hadn't had it done already. I'm glad I had it done, and I'm glad it's behind me. It's not an easy process to go through right now, I guess, like I said, that I'd do it again in a minute if I was faced with the same circumstances. [Irene]

No, my feelings were all right. I wasn't sorry I did it....I was never sorry I did it....Not at all. I haven't got a regret at all.... No, honestly, I just can't say enough that I would have it done. I've talked to so many women that would not ever have anything like this done. [Ingrid]

No, would I have changed, would I decide not to do it, no. No. Would I have done it earlier in my life? No, because I was too busy having kids. So, no, really not. [Other than the nipples, any regrets?] No. [Meredith]

But, I've never for a second regretted my decision...No, absolutely none...I'd say go with your gut, and I don't regret. I do not regret what I did at all. I just wish I never had to go through the whole thing, and I wish I still had my breasts. But I don't want fake ones, because I'm just afraid they're just going to look awful. [Julia]

So, would I have done it again? I would do it again. But, you know, it's not easy...I mean, in general, I don't regret it, I mean but there are times when you just, you know...[Any regrets?] No, no, no, no, not at all. [Harriet]

I have no regrets having the surgery, none whatsoever. I would recommend it to anybody that has any kind of history that really feels that they want to beat this. It's their own personal thing, but I wouldn't have a problem trying to talk anybody into having it to chase the cancer. No, I think it was clean cut. In fact, when I made the decision and had a [surgery] date, I felt very good about it. I wasn't at all apprehensive, nervous. I was, "This is good" . . . I don't feel any different. No. Don't regret it at all. . . . [Vicky]

On a scale of one to ten, I'm going to say a ten, because, I think, if I went back to do it now, I don't think I'd change a single thing. [Joyce]

I think I've had a fairly simple-minded view of all of this. I've been very constant and steady in my feelings of relief and satisfaction with having made the decision. I honestly don't feel like I've regretted it for a minute in my life. And I didn't regret it at that time or any time since then. I think I felt just really relieved, and I do think that part of it was watching my sister die. I mean, you know, I've never gotten very far away from that. So, it has always felt like a decision that I've been grateful to have had a chance to make, and I'm very comfortable with it. [Sandra]

Well, life goes on. Your life will go on, and you'll be there to enjoy it! [Chantal]

CHAPTER 11

Long Views on Prophylactic Mastectomy

Prophylactic mastectomy (PM) is a procedure which has at times been called "disfiguring" and "barbarous" and has been deemed by some—including some physicians—as unacceptable. However, with more information about the substantial benefits of PM in risk reduction for women who face greatly increased risk of breast cancer because of inherited genetic factors, there has been growing acceptance that PM is, for some women, an important option which greatly reduces their significant breast cancer risk. As the previous chapters and words of women who have undergone PM have revealed, many women find this option not to be easy, but to be very satisfying and rebalancing, allowing them to focus on life issues other than fear of breast cancer. Genetic advances now allow us to test a woman considering PM to determine whether she is actually in this high risk group or if she has only a general population breast cancer risk. Unfortunately, even genetic testing does not provide the clear answers in all circumstances that we would ideally have when a decision of this magnitude is to be made. But for many women who have a 50/50 chance of inheriting a mutation known to have caused breast cancer in close family members, this piece of the puzzle in the decision about PM can be achieved with a simple blood test. However, receiving a positive result on a test for a *BRCA1/2* mutation is only the beginning of the decision making which allows a woman to decide if PM is a reasonable option for her.

If you are a woman who is currently considering PM, we hope that the previous chapters have given you a context for thinking through your own circumstances, values, needs, fears, and tolerances. There is no single "right" answer as to whether PM is the right decision for you Coming to that decision requires a balance of what risks you can accept and live with, what changes in your body are acceptable or not, and what tolerance you have for repeated screening measures and potentially prolonged uncertainty about cancer. Because people naturally differ greatly in these qualities and because of the differences in women's personal and familial experience of breast cancer, there is no immediate answer to the question of whether PM is right for you or not. Only you can find that answer, often after considerable soul-searching and sometimes gut-wrenching consideration of the issues. You will find an answer and the more energy you give to a consideration of the pros and cons, the more likely it is that you will find peace and satisfaction in your decision, whatever it is.

IS PM A REASONABLE TRADE-OFF OR A BARBAROUS DEAL WITH THE DEVIL?

It seems clear that many women who have chosen to undergo PM are not only satisfied with their decision, they are very satisfied. They no longer believe getting breast cancer is inevitable; they feel free of a family curse. They have worries about breast cancer affecting others in their family, but they do not really worry for themselves. They worry about possible ovarian cancer risks, but many women who know they are *BRCA1/2* mutation carriers have elected to have their ovaries removed prophylactically to reduce that risk as well.[1]

In the United States[2] and, interestingly, in other countries including China,[3] the percentage of high risk women choosing PM is closer to 20 to 25 percent. In some other countries, notably the Netherlands and Denmark,[4, 5] up to about half of the women who are offered PM because of high hereditary risk accept this surgery and the outcomes are similar to those of the sample whose reactions we have examined in depth in this book. A follow-up report from the Netherlands found the majority of post PM women expressing satisfaction, although complications and disappointment with reconstruction outcomes limited satisfaction for some women.[4] Issues about sexual functioning, body image, and femininity did affect quality of life after surgery, but nonetheless, 95 percent of the women felt they would opt again for PM.

Not all women see their way to eventually undergoing PM surgery, even high risk women. For these women, PM feels like it is upsetting a natural order of things, while taking away too much of their body for the benefits which may follow, and disrupting too much of their lives and sense of comfort with themselves for what are hypothetical risks, not current disease. Some women feel that PM goes beyond what anyone who is not ill should do to change their body. Many women find the uncertainties of surgical outcome and the necessity to undergo often repeated reconstructive or corrective surgeries to be unacceptable. Women at known high risk for breast cancer have the alternative option of enhanced screening with more frequent mammograms and breast MRIs and many feel these are more acceptable options for them than surgery. This choice allows women to match their own views and feelings with the medical options available to find the best solution for them personally.

HOW DO I KNOW IF PM WILL BE OKAY FOR ME?

A simple first question is to consider how much does worry about breast cancer affect or interfere with your life. How much do you worry about getting or dying from breast cancer? Do you worry about dying before your young children have grown? How much anxiety do you feel about the uncertainties of repeated mammograms and other screening efforts to control your high risks for cancer? How often do you wish concern about breast cancer could be moved to a less prominent position in what you think or have to be vigilant about? If these are issues which trouble you, then you may find it helpful to consider PM. This would involve two steps. One step is gathering factual information about PM, talking to surgeons and plastic surgeons about what types of surgery and reconstruction would be possible with your body type and what would be involved in recovery. Try to determine the following: What are the risks of each surgical option? Would the surgery and reconstruction be paid for by your insurance?

The other step is the emotional "stocktaking" which is needed. How do you think you would feel about such surgery? What would it mean to you not to have breasts capable of sensation? Could you deal with the physical aspects of surgery? If you have never had surgery, this may be more difficult to assess. Is there relief in contemplating reduced breast cancer risk or is there more discomfort in thinking about significant changes in your body? Can you find women who have undergone PM to talk to about their experiences? Once you have some idea of what you truly feel, it would be important to talk to those closest to you, especially your sexual partner about what he or she thinks about the changes PM surgery would bring to your lives. Even though many women feel that this is their decision alone, talking with a partner may help you to decide what the impact of surgery would be on your life. What kind of support would you need to undergo surgery and is it available? Does it seem feasible, given your current life plans and responsibilities, to have surgery now or in the near future?

This is a significant decision and many women take years to make it.[6, 7] You may not want to think much about PM now, especially if you are young and just starting a family. On the other hand, some young women feel PM is necessary early in their lives to protect them from early onset hereditary breast cancer which has affected their family. With increasing numbers of women undergoing genetic testing, there are increasing numbers of young women who have been informed by their mothers at young ages (often while still minors) that they may have a high hereditary risk of developing breast cancer, so more of them will likely be considering the option of PM. As some of the women in this book have indicated, considerations about PM affect dating—when to tell, how to tell. Nonetheless, some young women decide it is more important to confront the demon of high breast cancer risk early and to struggle with how to talk to those they are dating about PM, rather than to continuing to be at such high risk.

ARE THERE INDICATIONS IT MIGHT NOT BE THE RIGHT ANSWER FOR ME?

If your first strong feeling about PM is that it is "off the charts" in terms of what any woman should do in response to knowing she is at high risk for breast cancer, it is likely that you will not—at least now—change your mind. Some of the women in our study group did find that time and life events—breast cancer diagnoses or deaths among close relatives or friends, or "close calls" with repeated biopsies which turned out to be negative but caused considerable anxiety—led them over a period of years to change their views. If you feel your breasts are very important to you, and that they are central features in your sense of femininity and attractiveness, and you do not simultaneously feel strong fears about breast cancer, this will likely mean that you will prefer the option of screening. If you have strong feelings about breastfeeding your children and are not yet finished with your childbearing, at least for now PM is not your option. For some women, it is comforting to know that PM will be available at some later time if they decide it is very difficult to live with high breast cancer risk. For now, however, they want to pursue other options. Other women simply feel that PM is not an option that they would ever consider.

We hope that reading about the prophylactic mastectomy experience of the 21 women in this study can help all women, even those who think it is not a highly likely choice for them, to know what is truly involved and how women have felt about this surgery. We hope that having presented real information about the PM experience has helped you to decide if this is an option you want to explore or think about more now, if this is an option you might consider at a later time, or if you are certain this surgery is not for you.

THE IMPACT OF PERSONAL EXPERIENCE: WHY THIS IS SUCH A CHALLENGING DECISION TO MAKE

Information about surgical or reconstructive procedures is not sufficient to make the essential decision about PM. Part of the reason why this is a challenging decision for many women is because the history of breast cancer in their families and their personal experience of the disease strongly affects their feelings about PM. It has become clear in this book and in the literature on genetic testing in general that personal experience carries enormous weight in determining the actions of women from high risk cancer families.[8] The decision whether to have PM brings up complex psychological issues. Feelings about the cancer experience of a mother (or grandmother or aunt), the experience of the woman considering PM herself during that time, and the eventual outcome all play a role in the decision making about PM and strongly influence the decision that is made.

The decision involves feelings about other sensitive aspects of a woman's life as well. For example, her sense of her own attractiveness; her comfort level in her intimate relationship or her worries about attracting a partner, if she is currently not in such a relationship; her feelings about her body generally and her breasts, in particular; her sense of herself as a mother and wife; her feelings about wanting or not wanting more children; whether breastfeeding in the future is important to her; her place in her family of origin and her relationships with parents and siblings; her feelings about aging and changed appearance with age. This is why talking with a psychologist or therapist is advisable before making the final decision—someone who can help the woman review her feelings and motivations and examine any aspects where there appear to be inherent conflicts, contradictions, or important issues which the woman may not have previously considered. Talking with a knowledgeable therapist can help a woman further refine her thinking about the pros and cons of PM and, if decided, about the timing of this surgery to fit best with her life plans and the impact of cancer fear on her daily experience.

MOTHERS AND MOTHERING

Mothers' bodies provide a little girl's first model for what the female body looks like and for how women relate to their bodies. When a mother has had breast cancer, the attitudes of her daughters are heavily influenced by changes in the mother's body and by how the mother reacted to them. Some of the women in our study had clearly maintained traumatizing images of early radical mastectomies which their mothers or grandmothers had undergone as treatment for cancer. These images served as a motivator—a reason to avoid breast cancer at all costs and to choose prospectively modern prophylactic mastectomy with, in most cases, reconstruction. Some of the women in our study had mothers who had strongly advocated for prophylactic mastectomy, advising their daughters to have a PM early on to prevent the chance of breast cancer. One woman dramed that her mother was approving of her PM as she awoke after surgery. Mothers' views are strongly influential, especially when a mother has died at an early age. The high incidence of maternal death from breast cancer in the group we interviewed is not a coincidence. Future in-depth interviews of women as they make their decisions could focus even more centrally on the influence of the mother and the mother's cancer experience on the daughter's decision making.

Among the women we interviewed, their own mothering played a central role in their decisions. Many seemed to feel that being a good mother demanded that they take every possible step to keep themselves alive in order to avoid their own mother's fate of developing breast cancer with the inherent risk of early death. This provided a model of significant sacrifice and proactive taking control over cancer risk for the sake of their children. It will be of great interest to see going forward how the next generation of women at high breast cancer risk interpret their mothers' experience and its implications for their expectations of themselves as they, in turn, become mothers.

One of the women we interviewed had had a grandmother who had undergone PM several decades before it was a recommended option and this seemed to help her to think of PM as a normalizing reaction to hereditary risk. Another woman who had undergone PM after the death of her sister from breast cancer worried that her daughter might be lulled into a false sense of security, if she turned out to be a mutation carrier since she would be unlikely to experience her mother being diagnosed breast cancer following the mother's PM.

HOW IS A PHYSICIAN TO KNOW WHAT TO ADVISE?

Information about levels of hereditary cancer risk and about surgery and reconstructive options are, of course, critical for women to have. It is important that this information be provided in ways which allow the woman to understand what her likelihood is of developing breast and ovarian cancer over her lifetime and why some surgical options are open to her while others are not. It should be clear to the woman that there are pros and cons of all approaches and what they are, but that she also be made aware that she is both free to seek other opinions and that the final decision is hers alone. Medical professionals can also provide information concerning the evolution of breast cancer treatment in recent decades and how it continues to improve. This may help some women decide that their fears of exactly repeating their mother's and/or grandmother's experiences of breast cancer are unrealistic. Some women may also need to separate out what they remember as very disfiguring mastectomy surgery of a relative in past decades from that which they could expect if they choose PM today. Nonetheless, breast cancer continues to be fatal in some cases, so complete reassurance is not possible.

How can medical professionals help women making these decisions about PM? Many want to help, but beyond giving the woman the necessary medical information and telling her that this is a highly personal decision and advising her to take time to make it, they are often unsure of other steps. There may be some additional ways medical professionals can consider adding to their own roles in women's decision making. One is to consider some of their biases about who would or would not consider PM and to realize that some of what we have believed may be less predictive as more women come to their genetic information and this decision earlier in their lives. For example, we assumed that most young, unmarried women would not want to make a decision for PM surgery. However, depending on whether the young woman has experienced the death of her mother from breast cancer and/or may have known about the possibility of hereditary predisposition and PM for some time, there may in the years to come more young women willing to undergo PM. We are encountering a new generation of young women whose mothers had genetic testing in the last 15 years for *BRCA1/2*. We know from research studies that many of these women shared their genetic test results with their minor children, often shortly after they got their results.[9, 10] This emerging group of young, high-risk women have grown up knowing more about hereditary cancer risk than women in previous generations and possibly also about the risk-reducing options available to mutation carriers. They are likely to have higher chances of having family members who made a decision for PM and, thus, many are more likely to have firsthand knowledge of this procedure and its impact. This may alter the way young woman make their decisions about PM in the years to come.

Medical professionals can also raise questions which a women considering PM might ask. They can also suggest the support of a psychologist or therapist to help the woman consider her. (See "The Role of Psychological Consultation" below). The professional might encourage the woman to contemplate the question "How important are your breasts to you?" The narratives we gathered showed that many women who were willing to undergo PM had some disinvestment in their breasts which made their surgical removal "easier." For some of these women, the disinvestment was tied to their family history of breast cancer and their feeling that their breasts were "time bombs," or enemies threatening the woman's life. Other women felt that their breasts had been too large for their bodies or that they were "in the way" for many years prior to consideration of PM.

Other aspects of the woman's identity may affect her decision-making. For example, transgender women at high hereditary risk may see the medical rationale to remove their breasts because of high breast cancer risk as fitting well with their own wish to be devoid of breasts in order to achieve greater congruence between their psychological sense of their gender and their body configuration. At the other end of the continuum of attachment to one's breasts may be women who feel that, in spite of knowing that breasts are not all there is to femininity, feel their breasts are their best feature, an essential part of who they are and what makes them attractive to others, and allows them to feel attractive themselves. These feelings may all strongly influence the acceptability or unacceptability of PM.

BREAST IMPORTANCE OVER TIME

We know little of how women's feelings about their breasts develop and change over time. Clearly, from our interviews there are vast differences in how the women felt about their own natural breasts; some felt that their breasts had been a source of great pleasure while others associated pain and fear with breasts. Given the predominant role breasts play in games of sexual attraction, especially as portrayed in the media, the message is strongly conveyed in our society that women's breasts are important. Those women in our study who felt otherwise had often had life experiences which relabeled breasts as sources of worry and imminent life threat. Their prior disinvestment in their breasts appeared to make their PM decision easier. We do not know, however, the extent to which somewhat older women's higher acceptance of PM is due to diminished sense of the need for their breasts— they have an established mate and have grown children so breastfeeding is not a concern—or if it is simply related to greater fear of breast cancer as they approach the ages at which others in their family have been diagnosed. Future studies, especially longitudinal studies with young women as they decide about PM, will help us to answer these questions and offer improved guidance about the discussions which can help women decide about their own breast investment and its characteristics and limits.

Mothers of young children often think about PM as a way of ensuring that they will be there to raise their children. However, this is not true of all young mothers and the time frame in which they are willing to undergo PM may be quite different for different women. Not being able to pick up a small child for a period after surgery may make one mother wait to have PM, while another may want to have surgery as soon as possible due to deep-seated fears.

Medical professionals may also help women establish social connections with others who have undergone PM. Keeping a record of patients willing to talk to women considering PM, and matching women by some of their prominent demographic characteristics (married/single, have children, had mother with breast cancer, age, sexual orientation, etc.) and characteristics of the proposed surgery may be a time-consuming, but it can be enormously helpful, according to the women we interviewed. Allowing women to talk to those for whom surgical recovery was relatively easy and for whom it was complicated will also help women to make realistic choices.

What is the physician responsibility vis-à-vis the woman and her decision-making? Emiel Rutgers, a Dutch surgeon, recently talked about how, when he discusses PM with a woman with a high hereditary risk for breast cancer, he has to be sure that they have several long conversations before she makes a decision.[11] Then he says, "I have to look the woman in the eye and look her partner in the eye before I know if she really wants to do this." Rutgers feels strongly that his job is to restrain a woman's enthusiasm until he is sure she has fully considered all the major ramifications of surgery. In the medical literature, some of the few reports of women who had regret following surgery were those who felt their surgeon had been the one who made the decision, not they themselves.[12] It is likely that at different times medical professionals play alternating roles. They sometimes encourage a woman to consider PM if she is having difficulty coping with breast cancer fear or enhanced screening and at other times, they assist a woman who seems to be rushing to surgery to take more time to consider the fit between PM surgery and her own attitudes and feelings.

Surgeons and plastic surgeons, even if they do spend considerable time with a woman deciding about PM, do not have the time or training to fully explore and evaluate a woman's life experience and its relationship to this decision. For these reasons, it is important that physicians and surgeons ensure that a psychologist, social worker, or psychiatrist is available, preferably as an integrated part of their clinic, to help women process the issues which are unique to her as she makes her decision. Women in our study told us that they preferred an integrated approach where all or most women consulting about PM saw the psychologist as a routine part of the approach to decision making or to surgery.[13] This helped them to feel that the referral did not indicate that the doctor felt there was anything wrong with them or with their thought process related to their decision. He or she felt it was a highly emotional and individual decision and that seeing a psychologist was a service they offered to help women explore their unique weighing of the issues prior to surgery.

THE ROLE OF PSYCHOLOGICAL CONSULTATION

Some medical clinics suggest such psychology visits routinely and have psychologists easily available who are experienced in helping women with these decisions. Contrary to what some women believe, psychologists in this setting do not have preconceived notions about what decision the woman should reach, but are there to help her make or confirm the best decision for herself, recognizing that no one decision is right for all women. Women in our study have told us that while a few actually saw a psychologist as part of their decision making process, many wished they had. Even for women who feel sure that they want PM surgery, it is often helpful to have someone outside of your immediate family with whom to go over your reasons, to say out loud what you hope to achieve, what your fears are, and what you think it will be like to wake up from the procedure with your breasts removed. This kind of rehearsal can help with the subsequent coping process.

It may be more difficult than initially imagined to examine how much worry about breast cancer is affecting a particular woman. Women in our study told us that they only later realized the level of depression or anxiety related to breast cancer that they had been experiencing before surgery; talking with a psychologist or therapist may make this depression or anxiety more apparent to all concerned. The psychological consultation may also provide a place to talk about the different options available now that were not available to previous generations of women in the family. For some women, this brings up difficult memories and sometimes, even a little guilt, about being able to evade breast cancer where others were not so fortunate. The psychologist or therapist can help a woman deal with these feelings which, in turn, can help her feel stronger about her decision, and able to go forward with energy and a sense of empowerment about having sorted through complex issues to come to a solid decision.

Talking with a psychologist or therapist can also allow a woman to think about how she and her partner can prepare for the surgery itself and for the changes it will bring to their sexual experience. Partners—and even women themselves—rarely talk aloud about what they will miss, what the woman's breasts have meant to their pleasure. In the context of a woman's decision making, partners often feel that they should keep such feelings to themselves, that they are selfish and would be seen as conveying a lack of caring about the woman's survival or comfort, or would seem to reduce their relationship to physical realities rather than to the integrated sexual and interpersonal complexity they share. Talking about such concerns can bring relief to both partners and can make them feel closer to each other as they each endure the losses which PM surgery inevitably brings. It may actually be helpful to the woman to hear how much the spouse or partner has enjoyed her breasts, to share the fear they each likely have about how they will feel about the woman's changed body, and their thoughts about how the lack of breasts or the reconstructed breasts will function in their future sexual encounters. For example, will it be okay for the man to find enjoyment in the reconstructed breasts if the woman does not have sensation and arousal as a result?

Opening lines of communication about all aspects of the couple's experience of the new breasts can help a woman and her partner feel less alone. If the partner has concern that surgery is an overreaction and is not necessary, it is better that the couple discuss these feelings before surgery rather than just trying to live with the consequences after it is a fait accompli. Particularly if the husband or partner has strong negative feelings about the woman undergoing PM, it will be important that he/she (in the case of lesbian partners) have a chance to air these views and that they talk about them before the woman makes a final decision and certainly, before the actual surgery. It may be helpful to have joint meetings with the psychologist or therapist and/or with the oncologist or surgeon so that they all can come to a place where they understand the decision which is ultimately made and the partner can support the wife in whatever she ultimately decides. Having these presurgery discussions will also make it more likely that the couple will resume useful, frank discussions about the changes after surgery. They will be less likely to fear that such conversations are off-limits or that talking about implicit losses with surgery would be destructive or hurtful rather than helpful and bonding. Acknowledging the losses does not take away from shared relief at the woman's reduced breast cancer risks.

INTEGRATING BODILY CHANGE: WHAT CONSTITUTES "WHOLENESS?"

The interviews in this book reveal that the women, all of whom had undergone PM, took different paths to redefining their bodies and that they all were satisfied or largely satisfied with their chosen paths. Some opted for no breast reconstruction and felt good about this decision, seeing the advantages of being able to go without a bra when they wished and feeling there was no physical impediment to feeling any lump which might develop in their chest at a very early point in time. Others took on the repeated surgeries of implants or opted for the surgical transformations of flap surgery—taking fat and muscle from elsewhere in the body to shape new breasts.

A number of the women talked about showing off their new breasts in ways which would often be considered inappropriate in other circumstances, taking off their tops in restaurant or workplace bathrooms to show off the surgical success in front of friends and colleagues, as one women described, "like a new car." Gradually with time, however, something changed for many of these women and this behavior no longer seemed appropriate. The new breasts had become part of their body and, thus, were not for display beyond their intimate partners. This process deserves more study so we can learn more about what changes and what determines how women come to feel about their new breasts. Are these feelings different for different forms of surgery or at different ages? What does the integration feel like emotionally? Some women have implied that with time, thoughts about their breasts could be relegated to the "back burner" so that they sometimes had to actively remember that the breasts they had were not their natural breasts. Our research was retrospective and cross-sectional, but it would be fascinating to follow women longitudinally through the PM process to better understand the steps in decision and adaptation and how women come to accept and think about their reconstructed bodies.

NIPPLES DO MATTER

Nipples are a focus in these narratives and other discussions about PM. As the sentient part of the breast, nipples are at the literal and figurative center of that which is lost in PM. Nipple-sparing PM surgery has been controversial, but is being reconsidered in recent medical reports.[14] Nipples contain breast tissue which, if not removed, could lead to breast cancer. Some surgeons have suggested that with women's strong feelings about their nipples, it might be preferable, even given the risk of residual breast tissue, to do nipple-sparing mastectomies (removing most of the breast tissue) rather than have the woman not undergo risk-reducing mastectomy at all. Other surgeons think that is an imprudent decision, given the remaining cancer risk. However, a recent effort in the Netherlands to do what is termed "nipple banking" shows the lengths to which women will go to preserve even a non-sentient nipple. Leonie A.E. Woerdeman, a Dutch plastic surgeon, recently reported on the high levels of satisfaction in most women who underwent this procedure.[15]

Nipple banking involves surgical removal in a fashion consistent with skin grafting of the nipple and the areola (or dark center of the breast), what is referred to as the nipple-areola complex (NAC), at the time the PM is initiated. The NAC is checked for cancer cells and is only preserved if it is cancer free. The NAC is then grafted elsewhere on the woman's body, often in the groin area where it remains, sometimes for as long as a year, while the rest of the PM reconstruction is completed. Then, the NAC is "replanted" onto the woman's reconstructed breast, allowing her to have her own original nipple with its known shape and coloring in most cases. The nipple is not attached to nerves as it once was and, hence, it is not capable of feeling. There are failure experiences in a minority of women in which reattachment is not possible or optimal. Rather to the surprise of the plastic surgeons doing nipple banking, the vast majority of the women undergoing nipple banking and reattachment felt that preserving their own nipple and areola went a long way towards making them feel whole and helped greatly with their postsurgical feelings of bodily integrity. Despite the fact that there were surgical complications and failures and that the implanted nipple in the woman's groin was often an impediment to optimal sexual functioning until it was reattached to the breast, women reported high levels of satisfaction with the nipple banking procedure. What does this teach us about women's conceptions of femininity and wholeness? The experience of nipple banking suggests again the idiosyncratic and personal nature of the experience of bodily wholeness in women undergoing PM. Satisfaction is not based on function, but familiarity. Breasts do not make a woman or define her femininity, but the ability to lose less of herself in the process of PM is highly valued. Women's views are the critical determinants of success once surgical competence is achieved. The narratives in this book point us in many interesting directions and further study of how women come to their feelings of psychological wholeness or reintegration will offer much of use to those advising women considering PM.

GENDER, SEXUALITY AND HEALTH: ARE THE EQUATIONS DIFFERENT FOR MEN AND WOMEN?

The argument has often been raised about whether men would be willing or would be asked to undergo a prophylactic procedure affecting an organ related to sexual functioning to reduce cancer risk. As one woman in our study noted:

> For me, I think, there's so many other ways that women—I mean, it's not like you're asking a man to have his penis off. There are so many other ways we enjoy sex, that, so, okay, fine, you don't get the same sexual stimulation from your breasts, but you can get it from all kinds of other places on your body. Do you follow what I'm saying? For me, I wonder how much that plays in their decision not to have their breasts off, because it isn't like they haven't started a family and they want to breastfeed their children. I can only think this is the thing that holds them up, because other than that, I can't find any explanation for it. I think it probably is a very, very big thing for other women, but it wasn't for me. [Joyce]

While there is not a direct equivalence of PM to asking a man, for example, to undergo prophylactic testicular or penile surgery, some feel that medicine would be unlikely to ask a healthy man to take off a sexual organ to prevent cancer were similar genetic information available to identify those at high hereditary risk of cancer in that organ. Women at high risk are asked to consider both PM and prophylactic oophorectomy, the removal of health ovaries (and usually Fallopian tubes) after their childbearing is complete. Prophylactic oophorectomy (PO) not only ends the option of having more pregnancies, but it also induces premature menopause, inducing hot flashes, the drying of many bodily surfaces including vaginal linings, which, in turn, affects sexual functioning. Sexual interest may be affected also by changes in hormonal balance. Women's lives and sexuality are changed by such surgeries,[16] although there are remedial measures which can reduce the effect and many women report relatively normal sexual functioning with time.

Are these reasonable tradeoffs to reduce risks of cancers which might never occur? Even with known *BRCA1/2* mutations which convey very high risks, the risks are not 100 percent. At least 15 percent of *BRCA1/2* mutation carriers never develop breast cancer and 60 percent or more of mutation carriers do not develop ovarian cancer. What makes women remove body parts under these circumstances? Some women in our study said that years after having surgery they revisited the possibility that they might never have been diagnosed with breast cancer without having had surgery, since the risk is not 100 percent. They said they felt that they might see those risks differently now than they did at the time of their decision, when breast cancer felt inevitable. However, this realization did not lead them to regret having had the surgery, but rather simply to acknowledge that how one looks at these issues and the equations of benefit and risk changes with time and experience.

SEXUALITY AND SAFETY

Many women would say that the PM decision did not focus so much on their concerns about their own attractiveness, but on their fears. Fear or cancer-related worry runs very high among women considering PM. Fear, in and of itself, is disfiguring and interfering and it can certainly interfere with sexual interest and enjoyment. Some of the women we interviewed even talked about how much more sexually available they felt postsurgery when they were not worried about dying young and when they could begin to envision a future without cancer. This may account for the fact that postmastectomy reports have included both negative and positive effects of surgery on sexual functioning.[4] Mothers of young children particularly spoke about their wish to be able to look ahead to events in their children's future without thoughts about whether they would be precluded from seeing the event because of breast cancer. Much of the satisfaction of PM is the relief in women's minds and the renewed anticipation that they will see their children grow up and that they will live to know their grandchildren.

Fear and security, then, are two ends of a continuum central to women's decisions about PM. The amount of threat determines the ease of decision making and the satisfaction with the actions one takes. Aron Ralston is well-known as the 27-year-old hiker who amputated his own arm when it was pinned under an immovable boulder on a mountain in Utah in 2003. After several days of trying to move the boulder and after he had drunk all the water he had with him, Ralston apparently was sanguine about his decision to save himself and stoic about any pain, cutting his arm off below the elbow, walking to get help and, when rescued, walking from the medical helicopter into the emergency room. What the women in our study said was essentially that they felt much like Aron, caught between a rock and a hard place, unable to move, but freed by the sacrifice of a body part which was threatening their continued existence.

Women in this study have traded physical wholeness for psychological freedom from fear. Removing their breasts also removed most of the fear of breast cancer which made them uncomfortable in the present and afraid of a future they thought they might not live to see. Their increased postsurgical comfort with their place in their life trajectory overshadowed physical discomfort, pain, and displeasure at transitional surgeries and bodily rearrangement. Even negative impact on sexual intimacy and body image took a back seat to satisfactions of having wrested control from the dangling uncertainties of high cancer risk. Action trumped waiting and watching for these women.

Genetic testing and attention to family cancer history alerted these women and their doctors to their high risks for breast cancer. In a society which views knowledge as a forerunner to power, there is an expectation that action should soon follow, especially when risk is up to 85 percent. Social focus on breast cancer no doubt sharpens focus on what can be done, not only to live a life with risk of breast cancer but to reduce that risk, if possible. For women choosing PM, watchful waiting to snare breast cancer at its earliest stage is insufficient and it does not relieve the nagging sense of passively waiting for cancer to occur. As more genes are found which predispose to more elevated disease risks, questions will arise about what people are willing to do to reduce other risks. The PM experience is instructive in that, if women have a choice of options, those who opt of their own accord for even quite extensive physical rearrangement, precipitating functional losses, may find satisfactions which others may find unacceptable. Trial and error about what matters (like nipple-banking) may help elucidate what improves satisfaction and reduces a sense of loss, even where loss (as in the loss of sensation) remains real. What do women want? Freedom from fear of high risk for frightening cancers and as much retention of self and naturally appearing form as possible.

IRONIES

There are a number of striking ironies in the stories of the women's PM surgeries, such as the elegant spareness of the Human Genome Project findings in comparison to the complexities of PM surgery and possible surgical reoperation and complication. Women saying they do not trust medicine and screening, so they opt for surgery instead, which is, of course, trusting a different branch of medicine. There is also the push by women for PM, especially before publication of the watershed articles, against doctors who saw such surgery as barbaric when women with cancer were being treated with lumpectomy. Then,

the reinvigoration of physician enthusiasm as clear data about the efficacy of PM emerged. Women having to push for something they
wanted which was, for some surgeons and physicians, too much medicine where they originally thought it did not belong, only to have the
women proved right, that the surgery they sought was, in fact, effective.
Women who chose not to undergo PM having biopsies as a result of
enhanced screening for breast cancer after their identification as
women at high hereditary risk for breast cancer growing tired of the
repeated fear as they waited for the biopsy result, leading them to opt
for PM. And finally, the wish for certainty on the part of everyone,
physicians and patients alike, and the great difficulty in truly achieving
it. Relative certainty, but no true 100 percent kind of guarantee. The
more we know, the more we realize what we do not know and cannot
control. Knowledge can be empowering indeed, but we do not yet have
sufficient knowledge to have the type of control we would want to have.

THE FUTURE

Genetic information and knowledge about the hereditary causes of
serious diseases like breast cancer offers the possibility that targeted
recommendation for those at increased risk can help people at high
risk avoid illness or detect it at the earliest stages through enhanced
screening. "Knowledge is Power" is a frequently heard statement
about why genetic information is worth having. Personalized medicine is a goal of this explosion of genetic new information about personal risk. While for many complex, common diseases, the goal of
personalized medicine is far from being reached, for women with
hereditary breast cancer in their family history, some aspects of personalized medicine are already available. Prophylactic mastectomy is
a way of drastically reducing the known elevated hereditary breast
cancer risk which threatens some women at earlier than usual ages
with developing breast cancer. Studies have shown that there is a more
than 90 percent risk reduction—a staggering figure in terms of other
types of cancer risk-reducing measures.

But the simple equation that "Knowledge is Power" overstates the
utility of this information about risk and risk reduction. Yes, women
have the option of electing PM, but this is not a no-brainer. It is not
like taking having a medicine to reduce risk, hopefully one with few
side effects. It is not like getting an injection or eating a certain food
to achieve 90+ percent risk reduction. PM is a life- and body-altering

surgery with many physical and emotional and interpersonal effects. And it raises questions for the woman trying to decide if it is right for her as well as broader social questions.

It is likely that PM as a prevention or risk-reduction method in women at high hereditary breast cancer risk will be supplanted in the future by other, easier, options. PM is an option during this phase in time, but it is likely that in the future there will be less invasive options available for mutation carriers and others at high risk to consider. They may be medications to turn off the deleterious effects of *BRCA1/2* mutations or therapy to repair the genetic mutations and their deleterious effects. There are currently a number of studies of what are called "parp inhibitors" which are being tested in both breast and ovarian cancer patients who are *BRCA1/2*–positive which show promise for treating tumors in mutation carriers with little or no side effects.[17] Whether these drugs or others can prevent the development of tumors in those at high risk who have not had cancer remains to be seen, but this will no doubt be evaluated in future studies.

A variety of methods of gene therapy may be available in the future to keep healthy those who are "lucky" enough to have clear genetic identification of their high breast cancer risk. How will women who have undergone PM feel when these treatments become available? Will they worry that they jumped too soon onto the surgical bandwagon? We do not, of course, know how quickly this area of research will advance, but we should probably take our best guess about the reaction of women who previously had PM from women who had PM surgery prior to the availability of genetic testing for breast cancer. Among those women, some subsequently found out that they were not indeed carriers of their familial mutation. These women did not express regret, but rather, sanguinely talked about having had to make their decision with the best information available at the time they needed to decide. They looked back at the years in between and the fears they had avoided by having undergone surgery and felt proud they had done what they could to minimize their risk. There is clearly a time and place historical frame around prophylactic mastectomy. It is for now and possibly for decades to come a reasonable, often very satisfying, option for women at high risk who carefully consider the personal pros and cons. With luck, the decision this book aims to help women make will become an unnecessary one for women with very high breast cancer risk in future generations. Until then, we hope that the narratives provided here make easier the decisions about how to reduce the risk of breast cancer for women at high hereditary risk.

APPENDIX A

Demographic Characteristics of Participants

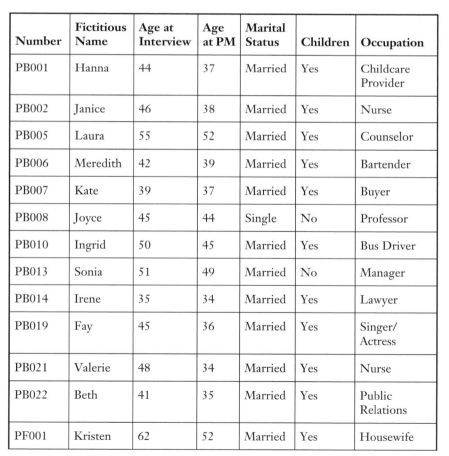

Number	Fictitious Name	Age at Interview	Age at PM	Marital Status	Children	Occupation
PB001	Hanna	44	37	Married	Yes	Childcare Provider
PB002	Janice	46	38	Married	Yes	Nurse
PB005	Laura	55	52	Married	Yes	Counselor
PB006	Meredith	42	39	Married	Yes	Bartender
PB007	Kate	39	37	Married	Yes	Buyer
PB008	Joyce	45	44	Single	No	Professor
PB010	Ingrid	50	45	Married	Yes	Bus Driver
PB013	Sonia	51	49	Married	No	Manager
PB014	Irene	35	34	Married	Yes	Lawyer
PB019	Fay	45	36	Married	Yes	Singer/ Actress
PB021	Valerie	48	34	Married	Yes	Nurse
PB022	Beth	41	35	Married	Yes	Public Relations
PF001	Kristen	62	52	Married	Yes	Housewife

(continued)

Number	Fictitious Name	Age at Interview	Age at PM	Marital Status	Children	Occupation
PF003	Alice	50	38	Married	Yes	Housewife
PM001	Vicky	55	50	Married	Yes	Nurse
PM002	Harriet	32	29	Married	Yes	Housewife
PM003	Rose	41	38	Married	Yes	Professor
PM005	Emily	49	46	Married	No	Nurse
PM008	Sandra	38	30	Married	Yes	College Administrator
PM011	Julia	46	44	Married	Yes	Nurse
PM012	Chantal	39	36	Married	Yes	Teacher

APPENDIX B

Interview Outline

ID Code #:_____   Time Started:_____

Interviewer:_____   Time Finished:_____

Date:_____   Total Time:_____

DECISION MAKING   Global Question #1: Could you please describe for me how you made your decision to have a prophylactic mastectomy (PM)? When did you first learn about PM, how did you think about it, who did you talk to, and how did you come to your final plan?

_____

_____

_____

_____

_____

_____

_____

_____

Probes (Ask only if not mentioned in narrative):

1a. What do you think you were hoping would be better about your life by undergoing this procedure? What were your personal aims or goals? How has it turned out?

_____

1b. How much were you worrying about cancer before surgery and how different, if at all, is your worry about cancer now?

1c. Presurgery: were you the kind of person who had mammograms and other screening tests right on time, put them off a little, or tended to avoid them?

1d. Were there some aspects of your own experience with cancer in your family which you were trying to avoid re-experiencing?

1e. Who, if anybody, had the most influence on your decision about PM? How did they influence you?

1f. Did your doctors make any recommendations about PM or not? How do you feel about the communication you had with your doctors about PM?

1g. When you were making your decision, what did you most want to know? Was any part of the information you got confusing? Did you have the information you wanted?

1h. As you were making your decision, did you talk to anyone who had had a PM? was that helpful?

_____
_____
_____

1i. Was it clear to you as you were making your decision that there was some residual risk of breast cancer even after having a PM? YES NO (If NO): Would knowing that have made a difference in your decision, do you think?

_____
_____
_____

(For All): How do you cope with knowing that?

_____
_____
_____

1j. Was your partner (if had one then) consulted? If yes, how was he/she involved? Did you find their involvement helpful or not? What was their reaction to your decision?

_____
_____
_____

1k. Do you think you are good at making medical decisions? Would you change anything about the way you approached this decision with the hindsight you now have?

_____
_____
_____

SURGICAL EXPERIENCE   Global Question #2: Could you please tell me what it was like to undergo your prophylactic mastectomy surgery? How did you feel going into the surgery and how did you find the recovery period?

_____
_____
_____
_____

_____
_____
_____
_____

Probes (Ask only if not mentioned in the narrative):

2a. Why did you choose to have the surgery at the time you did?

_____
_____
_____

2b. Did you have any hesitation about scheduling the surgery or keeping the appointment for surgery?

_____
_____
_____

2c. In the time leading up to the surgery, would you say that you had felt support or opposition or neither from the people closest to you? Were there any people close to you whom you did not tell about your impending surgery?

_____
_____
_____

2d. What was it like for you right after surgery? Was it different than you expected?

_____
_____
_____

2e. How did you feel about your body the first time the bandages were removed? What was helpful and what was not in adjusting to the way your body now looked?

_____
_____
_____

2f. Did you have any particular problems with pain management after surgery? Any complications?

_____
_____
_____

2g. What was the mobility of your arm like in the weeks and months following surgery?

_____
_____
_____

2h. What went into your decision about having/not having reconstruction? How did you decide about reconstruction?

_____
_____
_____

If had reconstruction: How did you decide when to have the reconstruction? Any problems with the reconstruction?

SURGICAL SEQUELAE/RECOVERY Global Question #3: What was it like for you after surgery? Was there an evolution in your feelings about your prophylactic mastectomy or did you feel pretty much the same about it from the time of surgery onward? If your feelings evolved, what were the turning points that resulted in your feeling differently about your surgery?

_____
_____
_____
_____
_____
_____
_____

Probes (Ask only if not discussed in the narrative):

3a. (If had reconstruction) What was it like emotionally to adjust to having a new breast?

_____

_____
_____

3b. How do you currently feel about your body?

_____
_____
_____

3c. Has your ability to play sports been affected at all?

_____
_____
_____

3d. Do you ever feel uncomfortable in dressing room or locker room situations because of your breasts?

_____
_____
_____

3e. How have your mastectomies affected your sense of your own sexual attractiveness? Your interest in or enjoyment of sex?

_____
_____
_____

FAMILY INVOLVEMENT   Global Question #4: Spouse/ Partner (For subjects with a spouse or partner): How did your partner react to your having had prophylactic surgery? Was there any change in your sexual relationship which you would attribute to your mastectomies? Did you see any change in your overall relationship, for better or worse?

_____
_____
_____
_____
_____
_____

Global Question #5: Children (For subjects with children): What did you tell your children at the time about your surgery and how have you talked about it with them since then, if at all?

_____
_____
_____
_____
_____
_____
_____
_____

Probes (Ask only if not discussed in narrative response):

5a. What have your children asked about your prophylactic surgery? How have you responded?

_____
_____
_____

5b. How important was having children to your decision to have pro-phylactic surgery?

_____
_____
_____

5c. Have you made suggestions to other family members about them having prophylactic mastectomies?

_____
_____
_____

MENTAL HEALTH INVOLVMENT   Global Question #6: How useful was it/would it have been to have a psychological consultation built into the presurgical consultation for PM?

_____
_____
_____
_____

_____

_____

_____

_____

Probes (Ask only if not discussed in narrative response):

6a. If you had services during the presurgical period, were they help-
    ful? In what way?

_____

_____

_____

6b. If you did not have mental health services during this period, did
    you consider talking to someone and if so, what prevented you from
    doing so?
    How do you think the counselor would have counseled/advised
    you?

_____

_____

_____

6c. Have you found mental health services useful at other times in
    your life?

_____

_____

_____

6d. How do you think you would have reacted if the surgeon you saw
    for your presurgical consultation had told you that speaking with a
    psychologist or other counselor had been a standard part of the
    presurgical work-up?

_____

_____

_____

6e. Would it have been helpful to be able to talk with a therapist after
    your surgery?

_____

_____

_____

6f. Do you think it would have been helpful if

a) the presurgical session had included roleplaying or rehearsal of your feelings following surgery,

b) or if any of the sessions had included

c) relaxation training or

d) a couple's session with you and your partner?

_____

_____

_____

6g. Would cost have been a barrier to seeing a counselor about PM?

_____

_____

_____

6h. Any suggestions about the ideal nature or timing or frequency of counselor involvement for people undergoing PM?

_____

_____

_____

SATISFACTION   Global Question #7: Overall, how satisfied are you with your prophylactic mastectomy? With your reconstruction (if applicable), with the emotional support you got from family, friends, professionals?

_____

_____

_____

_____

_____

_____

_____

_____

Probes (Ask only if not covered in narrative):

7a. How do you think it would be different for you today if you had not chosen to have a prophylactic surgery?

_____

_____

_____

7b. Did life come back to a place that you would call normal after your
    PM? If so, when would you say that occurred?

_____

_____

_____

7c. Any regrets?

_____

_____

_____

7d. Any suggestions for women considering PM?

_____

_____

                                           Time ended:_____

Interviewer Comments/Themes

_____

_____

_____

_____

_____

_____

_____

_____

APPENDIX C

Questions to Ask Medical Providers

How high is my breast cancer risk now?

Should I have genetic testing before I have a PM?

If the genetic testing is negative, but I still have a strong family history of breast cancer, should I still have a PM?

What other risks do I have and what can be done about them?

How much will PM reduce my breast cancer risk?

What are the alternatives to having a PM and how does the risk differ?

When should I have a PM?

What types of PM surgery are there and which types am I eligible for?

How painful is the surgery?

Will my insurance pay for it?

How long will I be in the hospital?

How many of these surgeries have you done? Is there anyone nearby who has done more?

For how long will I be unable to work? To pick up my children? To have sexual intercourse? (and anything else that is important to you.)

Do I need to see a plastic surgeon as well as a breast surgeon?

Is the reconstruction done right away or later?

Do they both need to work at the same hospital?

Will you be looking at my breast to see if it had any cancer in it?

What if you find any cancer?

What types of reconstruction are there?

How high is the complication rate with each method?

How long will each take?

What kind of clothes can I or can't I wear after surgery?

Are there sports or forms of exercise I won't be able or won't be advised to do after surgery?

What will happen to my breasts once they are removed? (optional)

What kind of surveillance will I need after the surgery?

Does reconstruction interfere with any of the surveillance? If I have reconstruction, will you be able to find a cancer if I ever develop one in my chest?

How should I explain this to my family—my husband, my mother and siblings, my children?

Is there anything in the pipeline now that might become available soon that would make having a PM unnecessary?

Bibliography

CHAPTER 1

1. Patricia Jasen, "Breast cancer and the language of risk, 1750–1950," *Social History of Medicine* 15 (2002): 17–43, doi: 10.1093/shm/15.1.17.

2. Sakorafas, G. H. and Michael Safioleas, "Breast cancer surgery: An historical narrative. Part III. From the sunset of the 19th to the dawn of the 21st century," *European Journal of Cancer Care* 19 (2010): 145–166, doi: 10.1111/j.1365-2354.2008.01061.x.

3. Skytte et al., "Risk reducing mastectomy and salpingo-oophorectomy in unaffected BRCA mutation carriers: Uptake and timing," *Clinical Genetics* 77 (2010): 342–349, doi: 10.1111/j.1399.0004.2009.01329.x.

4. Miki et al., "A strong candidate for the breast and ovarian cancer susceptibility gene BRCA1," *Science* 266 (1994): 66–71, doi: 10.1126/science.7545954.

5. Wooster et al., "Identification of the breast cancer susceptibility gene BRCA2," *Nature* 378 (1995): 789–792, doi: 10.1038/378789a0.

6. Ford, Deborah and Douglas F. Easton, "Risks of cancer in BRCA1 mutation carriers," *Lancet* 343 (1994): 692–695, doi: 10.1016/s0140-6736(94)91578-4.

7. Struewing et al., "The risk of cancer associated with specific mutations of BRCA1 and BRCA2 among Ashkenazi Jews," *New England Journal of Medicine* 336 (1997): 1401–1408, doi: 10.1056/NEJM199705153362001.

8. Easton et al., "Breast and ovarian cancer incidence in BRCA1-mutation carriers," *American Journal of Human Genetics* 56 (1995): 265–271, PMID: 7825587.

9. Fordet al., "Genetic heterogeneity and penetrance analysis of the BRCA1 and BRCA2 genes in breast cancer families," *American Journal of Human Genetics* 62 (1998): 676–689, doi: 10.1086/301749.

10. Howlader et al., eds. "SEER Cancer Statistics Review, 1975–2008a," National Cancer Institute, Bethesda, MD, http://seer.cancer.gov/

csr/1975_2008/, based on November 2010 SEER data submission, posted to the SEER website, 2011.

11. The Breast Cancer Linkage Consortium, "Cancer risks in *BRCA2* mutation carriers," *Journal of the National Cancer Institute* 91 (1999): 1310–6, doi: 10.1093/jnci/91.15.1310.

12. Thompson, Deborah and Douglas F. Easton for the Breast Cancer Linkage Consortium, "Cancer incidence in *BRCA1* mutation carriers," *Journal of the National Cancer Institute* 94 (2002): 1358–1365, doi: 10.1093/jnci/94.18.1358.

13. Abeliovich et al., "The founder mutations 185delAG and 5382insC in BRCA1 and 6174delT in BRCA2 appear in 60% of ovarian cancer and 30% of early-onset breast cancer patients among Ashkenazi women," *American Journal of Human Genetics* 60 (1997): 505–514.

14. Patricia Tonin, "The limited spectrum of pathogenic *BRCA1* and *BRCA2* mutations in the French Canadian breast and breast ovarian cancer families, a founder population of Quebec," *Canadian Bulletin of Cancer* 93 (2006): 841–846.

15. Metcalfe et al., and the Hereditary Breast Cancer Clinical Study Group, "International variation in rates of uptake of preventive options in BRCA1 and BRCA2 mutation carriers," *International Journal of Cancer* 122 (2008): 2017–2022, doi: 10.1002/ijc.23340.

16. Friebel et al., "Bilateral prophylactic oophorectomy and bilateral prophylactic mastectomy in a prospective cohort of unaffected BRCA1 and BRCA2 mutation carriers," *Clinical Breast Cancer* 7 (2007): 875–882, doi: 10.3816/CBC.2007.n.053.

17. Phillips et al., "Risk-reducing surgery, screening and chemoprevention practices of BRCA1 and BRCA2 mutation carriers: a prospective cohort study," *Clinical Genetics* 70 (2006): 198–206, doi: 10.1111/j.1399-0004.2006.00665.x.

18. Lostumbo, Liz, Nora E. Carbine, and Judi Wallace, "Prophylactic mastectomy for the prevention of breast cancer," *Cochrane Database of Systematic Reviews* 11 (2010): Art. No.: CD002748, doi: 10.1002/14651858.CD002748.pub3.

19. Hartmann et al., "Efficacy of bilateral prophylactic mastectomy in women with a family history of breast cancer," *The New England Journal of Medicine* 340 (1999): 77–84, doi: 10.1056/NEJM199901143400201.

20. Gail et al., "Projecting individualized probabilities of developing breast cancer for white females who are being examined annually," *Journal of the National Cancer Institute* 81 (1989): 1879–1886, doi:10.1093/jnci/81.24.1879.

21. Meijers-Heijboer et al., "Breast cancer after prophylactic bilateral mastectomy in women with a BRCA1 or BRCA2 mutation," *New England Journal of Medicine* 345 (2001): 159–164, doi: 10.1056/NEJM200107193450301.

22. Eisen, Andrea and Barbara L. Weber, "Prophylactic mastectomy for women with *BRCA1* and *BRCA2* mutations–Facts and controversy," *New England Journal of Medicine* 345 (2001): 207–208, doi: 10.1056/NEJM 200107193450309.

23. Rebbeck et al., "Bilateral prophylactic mastectomy reduces breast cancer risk in BRCA1 and BRCA2 mutation carriers: The PROSE study group," *Journal of Clinical Oncology* 22 (2004): 1055–1062, doi: 10.1200/ JCO.2004.04.188.

24. Geiger et al., "A population-based study of bilateral prophylactic mastectomy efficacy in women at elevated risk for breast cancer in community practices," *Archives of Internal Medicine* 165 (2005): 516–520, doi: 10.1001/archinte.165.5.516.

25. Jemal et al., "Cancer statistics, 2010," *CA Cancer Journal for Clinicians* 60 (2010): 277–300, doi: 10.3322/caac.20073.

26. K. Offit, *Clinical Cancer Genetics: Risk Counseling and Management*, New York: Wiley-Liss, 1998.

27. Julian-Reynier et al., "Time to prophylactic surgery in BRCA1/2 carriers depends on psychological and other characteristics," *Genetic Medicine* 12 (2010): 801–807, doi: 10.1097/GIM0b013e3181f48d1c.

28. Ray Jessica A., Lois J. Loescher and Molly Brewer, "Risk-reduction surgery decisions high-risk women seen for genetic counseling," *Journal of Genetic Counseling* 14 (2005): 473–484, doi: 10.1007/s10897-005-5833-5.

29. Ackermann et al., "Acceptance for preventive genetic testing and prophylactic surgery in women with a family history of breast and gynaecological cancers," *European Journal of Cancer Prevention* 15 (2006): 474–479, doi: 10.1097/01.cej.0000220628.62610.ea.

30. Bresser et al., "Who is prone to high levels of distress after prophylactic mastectomy and/or salpingo ovariectomy?" *Annals of Oncology* 18 (2007a): 1641–1645, doi: 10.1093/annonc/mdm274.

31. Tan et al., "Standard psychological consultations and follow up for women at increased risk of hereditary breast cancer considering prophylactic mastectomy," *Hereditary Cancer in Clinical Practice* 7 (2009), doi: 10.1186/ 1897-4287-7-6.

32. Uyei et al., "Association between clinical characteristics and risk-reduction interventions in women who underwent BRCA1 and BRCA2 testing: a single-institution study," *Cancer* 107 (2006): 2745–2751, doi: 10.1002/ cncr.22352.

33. van Dijk et al., "Decision making regarding prophylactic mastectomy: Stability of preferences and the impact of anticipated feelings of regret," *Journal of Clinical Oncology* 14 (2008): 2358–2363, doi: 10.1200/ JCO.2006.10.5494.

34. Borgen et al., "Patient regrets after prophylactic mastectomy," *Annals of Surgical Oncology* 5 (1998): 603–606, doi: 10.1007/BF02303829.

35. Stefanek et al., 1995. "Predictors of and satisfaction with bilateral prophylactic mastectomy," *Preventive Medicine* 24 (1995): 412–419, doi: 10.1006/pmed.1995.1066.

36. Bresser et al., 2006. "Satisfaction with prophylactic mastectomy and breast reconstruction in genetically predisposed women." *Plastic and Reconstructive Surgery* 117: 1675–1682, doi: 10.1097/01.prs.0000217383.99038.f5.

37. Frost et al., "Long-term satisfaction and psychological and social function following bilateral prophylactic mastectomy," *Journal of the American Medical Association* 284 (2000): 319–324, doi: 10.1001/jama.284.3.319.

38. Josephson, U., M. Wickman, and K. Sandelin, "Initial experiences of women from hereditary cancer families after bilateral prophylactic mastectomy: a retrospective study," *European Journal of Surgical Oncology* 26 (2000): 351–356, doi: 10.1053/ejso.1999.0897.

39. Lodder et al., "One year follow-up of women opting for presymptomatic testing for BRCA1 and BRCA2: Emotional impact of the test outcome and decisions on risk management (surveillance or prophylactic surgery)," *Breast Cancer Research and Treatment* 73 (2002): 97–112, doi: 10.1023/A:1015269620265.

40. Metcalfe, Kelly A., John L. Semple, and Steven A. Narod, "Satisfaction with breast reconstruction in women with bilateral prophylactic mastectomy: A descriptive study," *Plastic and Reconstructive Surgery* 114 (2004): 360–362, doi: 10.1097/01.PRS.0000131877.52740.0E.

41. Spear et al., "Prophylactic mastectomy and reconstruction: clinical outcomes and patient satisfaction," *Journal of Plastic and Reconstructive Surgery* 122 (2008): 340–347, doi: 10.1097/PRS.0b013e318177415e.

42. Zion et al., "Reoperations after prophylactic mastectomy with or without implant reconstruction," *Cancer* 98 (2003): 2152–2160, doi: 10.1002/cncr.11757.

43. Barton et al., "Complications following bilateral prophylactic mastectomy," *Journal of the National Cancer Institute Monographs* 35 (2005): 61–66, doi: 10.1093/jncimonographs/lgi039.

44. Drazen et al., "Bilateral breast reconstruction with DIEP flaps: 4 years' experience," *Journal of Plastic and Reconstructive and Aesthetic Surgery* 61 (2008): 1309–1315, doi: 10.1016/j.bjps.2007.06.028.

45. Hatcher, Mai Bebbington, Lesley Fallowfield, and Roger A'Hern, "The psychosocial impact of bilateral prophylactic mastectomy: Prospective study using questionnaires and semi-structured interviews," *British Journal of Medicine* 322 (2001): 76–79, doi: 10.1136/bmj.322.7278.76.

46. Van Oostrum et al., "Long-term psychological impact of carrying a *BRCA1/2* mutations and prophylactic surgery: a 5-year follow-up study," *Journal of Clinical Oncology* 21 (2003): 3867–3874, doi: 10.1200/JCO.2003.10.100.

47. Bresser et al., "The course of distress in women at increased risk of breast and ovarian cancer due to an (identified) genetic susceptibility who

opt for prophylactic mastectomy and/or salpingo-oophorectomy," *European Journal of Cancer* 43 (2007b): 95–103, doi: 10.1016/j.ejca.2006.09.009.

48. Wasteson et al., "High satisfaction rate ten years after bilateral prophylactic mastectomy–a longitudinal study," *European Journal of Cancer Care* 20 (2010): 508–513, doi: 10.1111/j.1365-2354.2010.01204.x.

49. Gahm, Jessica, Marie Wickham, and Yvonne Brandberg, "Bilateral prophylactic mastectomy in women with inherited risk of breast cancer: Prevalence of pain and discomfort, impact on sexuality, quality of life and feelings of regret two years after surgery," *The Breast* 19 (2010): 462–469, doi: 10.1016/j.breast.2010.05.003.

50. Metcalfe et al., "Predictors of quality of life in women with a bilateral prophylactic mastectomy," *The Breast Journal* 11 (2005): 65–69, doi: 10.1111/j.1075-122X.2005.21546.x.

51. Isern et al., "Aesthetic outcome, patient satisfaction, and health-related quality of life in women at high risk undergoing prophylactic mastectomy and immediate breast reconstruction." *Journal of Plastic, Reconstructive and Aesthetic Surgery* 61 (2008): 1177–1187, doi: 10.1016/j.bjps.2007.08.006.

52. Amy McGaughry, "Body image after bilateral prophylactic mastectomy: an integrative literature review," *Journal of Midwifery and Women's Health* 51 (2006): e45–49, doi: 10.1016/j.jmwh.2006.07.002.

53. Maxwell et al., "Advances in nipple-sparing mastectomy: Oncological safety and incision selection," *Aesthetic Surgery Journal* 31 (2011): 310–319, doi: 10.1177/1090820X11398111.

54. Rozen W. M. and M. W. Ashton, "Improving outcomes in autologous breast reconstruction," *Aesthetic Surgery Journal* 33 (2009): 327–335, doi: 10.1007/s00266-008-9272-1.

55. Man, Li-Xing, Jesse C. Selber, and Joseph M. Serletti, "Abdominal wall following free TRAM or DIEP flap reconstruction: A meta-analysis and critical review." *Plastic and Reconstructive Surgery* 124 (2009): 752–764, doi: 10.1097/PRS.0b013e31818b7533.

56. Spear, Scott L. and M. Renee Jespersen, "Breast implants: saline or silicone?" *Aesthetic Surgery Journal* 30 (2010): 557–570, doi: 10.1177/1090820X10380401.

57. Rolnick et al., "What women wish they knew before prophylactic mastectomy," *Cancer Nursing* 30 (2007): 285–291, doi: 10.1097/01.NCC.0000281733.40856.c4.

58. Scott L. Spear, "Reoperations or revisions." *Plastic and Reconstructive Surgery* 119 (2007): 1943–1944, doi: 10.1097/01.prs.0000259187.49061.04.

59. Batista et al., "Coordinated prophylactic surgical management for women with hereditary breast-ovarian cancer syndrome." *Biomedical Central Cancer* 8 (2008): 101, doi: 10.1186/1471-2407-8-101. DOI: 10.1186/1471-2407-8-101.

60. De Leeuw, J. R., M. J van Vliet, and M. G. Ausems, "Predictors of choosing life-long screening or prophylactic surgery in women at high and

moderate risk for breast and ovarian cancer," *Familial Cancer* 7 (2008): 347–359, doi: 10.1007/s10689-008-9189-5.

CHAPTER 2

1. Press et al., "That's like chopping off a finger because you're afraid it might get broken: Disease and illness in women's views of prophylactic mastectomy," *Social Science Medicine* 61 (2005): 1106–1117, doi: 10.1016/j.socscimed.2005.01.012.

CHAPTER 3

1. Hartmann et al., 1999, "Efficacy of bilateral prophylactic mastectomy in women with a family history of breast cancer," *The New England Journal of Medicine* 340 (1999): 77–84, doi: 10.1056/NEJM199901143400201.
2. Meijers-Heijboer et al., "Breast cancer after prophylactic bilateral mastectomy in women with a BRCA1 or BRCA2 mutation," *New England Journal of Medicine* 345 (2001): 159–164, doi: 10.1056/NEJM200107193450301.
3. Friebel et al., "Bilateral prophylactic oophorectomy and bilateral prophylactic mastectomy in a prospective cohort of unaffected BRCA1 and BRCA2 mutation carriers," *Clinical Breast Cancer* 7 (2007): 875–882, doi: 10.3816/CBC.2007.n.053.

CHAPTER 5

1. Borgen et al., "Patient regrets after prophylactic mastectomy," *Annals of Surgical Oncology* 5 (1998): 603–606, doi: 10.1007/BR02303829.
2. Gahm, Jessica, Marie Wickham, and Yvonne Brandberg, "Bilateral prophylactic mastectomy in women with inherited risk of breast cancer: Prevalence of pain and discomfort, impact on sexuality, quality of life and feelings of regret two years after surgery," *The Breast* 19 (2010): 462–469, doi: 10.1016/j.breast.2010.05.003.
3. Spear et al., "Nipple-sparing mastectomy." *Plastic and Reconstructive Surgery* 123 (2009): 1665–1673, doi: 10.1097/PRS.0b013e3181a64d94.
4. Maxwell et al., "Advances in nipple-sparing mastectomy: oncological safety and incision selection," *Aesthetic Surgery Journal* 31 (2011): 310–319. doi: 10.1177/1090820X11398111.

CHAPTER 6

1. Hansen, Dorthe Marie, Henrik Kehlet, and Rune Gartner, "Phantom breast sensations are frequent after mastectomy," *Danish Medical Bulletin* 58 (2011): A4259.

CHAPTER 7

1. Daniel Kahneman, "A perspective on judgment and choice: mapping bounded rationality," *American Psychologist* 58 (2003): 697–720, doi: 10.1037/0003-066X.58.9.697.

2. Lapointe et al., "Incidence and predictors of positive and negative effects of BRCA1/2 genetic testing on familial relationships: A 3-year follow-up study," *Genetics in Medicine* (In press).

3. Smith et al., "Familial context of genetic testing for cancer susceptibility: Moderating effect of siblings' test results on psychological distress one to two weeks after *BRCA1* mutation testing," *Cancer Epidemiology, Biomarkers & Prevention* 8 (1999): 385–392.

4. Patenaude et al., "Sharing *BRCA1/2* test results with first-degree relatives: Factors predicting who women tell," *Journal of Clinical Oncology* 24 (2006): 700–706, doi: 10.1200/JCO.2005.01.7541.

CHAPTER 9

1. Marris, S., S. Morgan, and D. Stark, "Listening to patients: What is the value of age-appropriate care to teenagers and young adults with cancer?" *European Journal of Cancer Care* 20 (2011): 145–171, doi: 10.1111/j.1365-2354 .2010.01186.x.

2. Boothroyd, R. I. and E. B. Fisher, "Peers for progress: Promoting peer support for health around the world," *Family Practice* 27 Suppl 1 (2010): 62–68, doi: 10.1093/fampra/cmq017.

3. Hilfinger et al., "Embodied work: Insider perspectives on the work of HIV/AIDS peer counselors," *Health Care Women International* 30 (2009): 572–594, doi: 10.1080/07399330902928766.

CHAPTER 10

1. Wasteson er al., "High satisfaction rate ten years after bilateral prophylactic mastectomy–a longitudinal study," *European Journal of Cancer Care* 20 (2010), doi: 10.1111/j.1365-2354.2010.01204.x.

2. Spear et al., "Prophylactic mastectomy and reconstruction: clinical outcomes and patient satisfaction," *Journal of Plastic and Reconstructive Surgery* 122 (2008): 340–347. doi: 10.1097/PRS.0b013e318177415e.

CHAPTER 11

1. Lostumbo, Liz, Nora E. Carbine, and Judi Wallace, "Prophylactic mastectomy for the prevention of breast cancer," *Cochrane Database of Systematic Reviews* 11. No. CD002748 (2010), doi: 10.1002/14651858.CD002748.pub3.

2. Friebel et al., "Bilateral prophylactic oophorectomy and bilateral prophylactic mastectomy in a prospective cohort of unaffected BRCA1 and BRCA2 mutation carriers," *Clinical Breast Cancer* 7 (2007): 875–882. doi: 10.3816/CBC.2007.n.053.

3. Kwong et al., "Choice of management of southern Chinese BRCA mutation carriers," *World Journal of Surgery* 34 (2010): 1416–1426, doi: 10.1007/s00268-010-0477-5.

4. Bresser et al., "Satisfaction with prophylactic mastectomy and breast reconstruction in genetically predisposed women," *Plastic and Reconstructive Surgery* 117 (2006): 1675–1682, doi: 10.1097/01.prs.0000217383.90038.

5. Skytte et al., "Risk reducing mastectomy and salpingo-oophorectomy in unaffected BRCA mutation carriers: uptake and timing," *Clinical Genetics* 77 (2010): 372–349. doi: 10.1111/j.1399-0004.2009.01329.x.

6. Bradbury et al., "Uptake and timing of bilateral prophylactic salpingo-oophorectomy among BRCA1 and BRCA2 mutation carriers," *Genetics in Medicine* 10 (2008): 161–166, doi: 10.1097/GIM.0b013e318 163487d.

7. Julian-Reynier et al., "Time to prophylactic surgery in BRCA1/2 carriers depends on psychological and other characteristics," *Genetics in Medicine* 12 (2010): 801–807, doi: 10.1097/GIM.0b013e3181f48d1c.

8. Katapodi et al., "Predictors of perceived breast cancer risk and the relation between perceived risk and breast cancer screening: a meta-analytic review," *Preventive Medicine* 38 (2004): 388–402, doi: 10.1016/j.ypmed. 2003.11.012.

9. Tercyak et al., "Parent-child factors and their effect on communicating BRCA1/2 test results to children," *Patient Education and Counseling* 47 (2002): 145–153, doi: 10.1016/50738-3991(01)00192-6.

10. Bradbury et al., "How often do BRCA mutation carriers tell their young children of the family's risk for cancer? A study of parental disclosure of BRCA mutations to minors and young adults," *Journal of Clinical Oncology* 25 (2007): 3705–3711, doi: 10.1200/JCO.2006.09.1990.

11. Emiel Rutgers, Preventative surgery for breast cancer risk, Talk presented at the 12th International Meeting on Psychosocial Aspects of Hereditary Cancer, Amsterdam, the Netherlands, April 27–29, 2011.

12. Lodder et al., "One year follow-up of women opting for presymptomatic testing for *BRCA1* and *BRCA2*: Emotional impact of the test outcome and decisions on risk management (surveillance or prophylactic surgery)," *Breast Cancer Res. Treat.* 73 (2002): 97, doi: 10.1023/A: 1015269620265.

13. Patenaude et al., "Support needs and acceptability of psychological and peer consultation: attitudes of 108 women who had undergone or were considering prophylactic mastectomy," *Psycho-Oncology* 17 (2008): 831–843, doi: 10.1002/pon.1279.

14. Patrick et al., "Advances in nipple-sparing mastectomy: oncological safety and incision selection," *Journal of Aesthetic Surgery* 31 (2011): 310–319, doi: 10.1177/1090820X11398111.

15. Leonie A. E. Woerdeman, Immediate breast reconstruction and nipple banking in prophylactic mastectomy. Talk presented at the 12th International Meeting on Psychosocial Aspects of Hereditary Cancer, Amsterdam, the Netherlands, April 27–29, 2011.

16. Matloff Ellen T., Rachel E. Barnett, and Sharon L. Bober, "Unraveling the next chapter: sexual development, body image, and sexual functioning in female BRCA carriers," *Cancer* 15 (2009): 15–18, doi: 10.1097/PPO.0b013e31819585f1.

17. Annunziata, Christina M. and Susan E. Bates. "PARP inhibitors in BRCA1/BRCA2 germline mutation carriers with ovarian and breast cancer," *F1000 Biol Reports* 2 (2010): 10, doi: 10.3410/B2-10.

Index

About the Author

ANDREA FARKAS PATENAUDE, PhD, is a clinical and research psychologist who is Center for Cancer Genetics and Prevention Director of Psychology Research and Clinical Services in the Department of Psychosocial Oncology and Palliative Care at the Dana-Farber Cancer Institute Boston, Massachusetts. Dr. Patenaude is also an Associate Professor of Psychology in the Department of Psychiatry at Harvard Medical School, Boston. She received her undergraduate degree in Psychology from the University of Chicago and her doctorate from Michigan State University.

From the beginning of the era of genetic testing for hereditary cancer in the mid-1990s, Dr. Patenaude has been involved in studying psychological, physical, interpersonal, and psycho-sexual consequences of being a mutation carrier for a cancer predisposition gene. She has worked with patients from families affected with hereditary breast/ovarian cancer, colorectal cancer, Li-Fraumeni Syndrome, and other pediatric and adult hereditary cancers. Her interest in genetics and the family guide much of her work.

She is the author of *Genetic Testing for Cancer: Psychological Approaches to Helping Patients and Families* published in 2005 by APA Books as well as many peer-reviewed journal articles, book chapters, and editorials. Dr. Patenaude's research has been funded by the National Institutes of Health, the Department of Defense Breast Cancer Research Program, the American Cancer Society, and other government and private foundations. She has served on panels at the National Human Genome Research Institute, the Department of Defense Breast Cancer Research Program, the American Psychological Association, the National Coalition for Health Professional Education in Genetics, and other national and international groups interested in studying the human impact of genetic testing for cancer.